T0136358

Surgical and Anaesthetic Instruments for OSCEs

Surgical and Anaesthetic Instruments for OSCEs
A Practical Study Guide

Kelvin Yan

NIHR Academic Clinical Fellow, University of Oxford
Honorary Clinical Research Fellow, Imperial College London

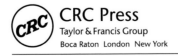

CRC Press
Taylor & Francis Group
Boca Raton London New York

CRC Press is an imprint of the
Taylor & Francis Group, an **informa** business

First edition published 2021
by CRC Press
6000 Broken Sound Parkway NW, Suite 300, Boca Raton, FL 33487-2742

and by CRC Press
2 Park Square, Milton Park, Abingdon, Oxon, OX14 4RN

ISBN: 978-0-367-35894-5 (hbk)
ISBN: 978-0-367-33050-7 (pbk)
ISBN: 978-0-429-34251-6 (ebk)

Typeset in Master Pass
by Deanta Global Publishing Services, Chennai, India

Contents

Part Two   Surgical Instruments

Preface

Surgical and Anaesthetic Instruments for OSCEs: A Practical Study Guide is intended for both undergraduate and postgraduate students and trainees of medical disciplines interested in learning the basic healthcare equipment that they may come across in the workplace. There are many instrument books in the market that either go into too much detail or do not explain the basics of these instruments in a concise manner. There are currently no publications that combine basic anaesthetic and surgical instruments in a single text. I therefore hope that the presentation of this book will fill this gap and stimulate interest and motivation in learning this subject matter.

I have developed the book in a question and answer format mimicking what it is like in an exam. I believe this will make one's learning more structured and focussed without going into minute detail. It is obviously impossible to encompass the entire syllabus of anaesthetic and surgical instruments in one textbook; this guide by no means pretends in any way that it serves this purpose. Rather, I want to cover the basic instruments that we use and see daily, explain them in a concise manner and help readers enjoy the process of learning something that will hopefully benefit their day-to-day job.

For those interested in learning more about the subject matter, I have included references for further reading. These are by no means comprehensive but serve to guide the reader's direction into further learning in a more detailed manner.

I believe that images and illustrations aid our learning tremendously, especially when it comes to anaesthetic and surgical instruments. Many students may have seen these instruments from afar but have never had the opportunity to examine them closely. The inclusion of illustrative images is therefore one of the strongest merits of this book. Much of the work would not have been possible without the contribution of the manufacturers and suppliers. Their generous contribution to the images has made illustrations of these instruments possible.

Another merit of this book is the accompanying explanations. I set out to explain the rationale, indications, contraindications and complications of the instruments, as opposed to merely listing them with names and intended functions. I believe this will aid readers in learning the instruments in a more well-rounded manner whilst covering "why-we-do-certain-things" in medicine. This approach, in my opinion, is paramount in learning medicine which requires flexible thinking rather than simply following protocols. It also ensures that readers will learn around the topic rather than purely memorise instrumental indications. As such, I hope this book will serve to motivate you in your training career in a different way.

Lastly and most importantly, I hope you will enjoy the book.

Author

Dr Kelvin Yan, MRCP, AICSM is an NIHR Academic Clinical Fellow, University of Oxford and an Honorary Clinical Research Fellow, Imperial College London.

Part One

ANAESTHETIC EQUIPMENT

AIRWAY

1

Endotracheal Tube

What Is This?

This is an endotracheal tube which is used to secure a definitive airway (Figure 1.1). It is inserted into the trachea to ventilate the patient. It has an inflatable cuff to prevent aspiration.

What Are the Indications?

Main indications are 1) ensuring airway patency for ventilation and 2) preventing aspiration. In an elective situation, these include any prolonged operations, excessive movement of the head and neck during surgery and situations where major intraoperative complications or risks of regurgitation/aspiration are likely. Indications in emergency situations include the inability of

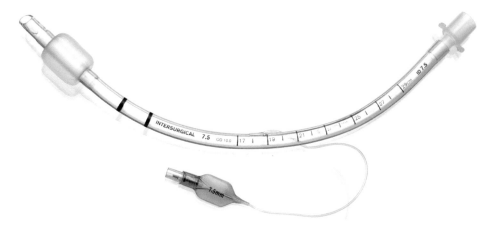

Figure 1.1   Endotracheal Tube. *Courtesy of Intersurgical Ltd.*

a patient to protect their airway and/or ventilate (reduced Glasgow Coma Scale [GCS], cardiac/respiratory arrest), inability of a conscious patient to adequately ventilate (severe/life-threatening asthma attacks, severe chest infections, neuromuscular complications from conditions such as myasthenic crisis and Guillain-Barré Syndrome) and any potential obstruction of the airway such as anaphylaxis and respiratory burns.

What Are the Contraindications?

Severe trauma or airway obstruction proximal to the point at which the tube will be passed (pharyngeal foreign body, massive swelling of the pharynx). Special care must be taken in cases of cervical spine injuries where complete immobilisation is needed.

Do You Know of Any Complications of Using This Device?

Damage to the lips, teeth and oropharynx are not uncommon. Over-inflation of the cuff may cause high pressure on the tracheal wall leading to ischaemia whereas insufficient inflation may lead to a circuit leak. Misplacement/dislodgement of the endotracheal tube may lead to hypoxia and death. One-lung intubation as a result of the tube going too far can also lead to inadequate ventilation.

Laryngeal Mask Airway (LMA)

What Is This?

This is a laryngeal mask airway (Figure 1.2). It is used for supporting the airway sparing tracheal intubation. It was developed by a British anaesthetist, Dr Archie Brain, in the 1980s. It is inserted orally and sits in the hypopharynx against the upper oesophageal sphincter at the C6/C7 level.

What Are the Indications?

It is mainly used for inhalational anaesthesia. It is also used for maintaining the airway in unforeseen circumstances such as managing the airway in emergency situations when intubation is difficult or when expertise for intubation is lacking.

What Are the Contraindications?

LMAs should not be used when a definitive airway is indicated. Examples include perioperative airway management when there is a risk of aspiration, muscle relaxation is needed and the prone position during surgery.

Do You Know of Any Complications of Using This Device?

Laryngospasm is a major complication of LMA during surgery. Other complications include nausea, vomiting, arytenoid dislocation, vocal cord paralysis and a sore throat. Cranial nerve injuries are uncommon but can include the lingual, recurrent laryngeal and hypoglossal nerves.

How Many Types of LMA Do You Know Of?

Supreme LMAs, flexible LMAs, i-gels.

i-gel

What Is This?

This is an i-gel which is a single-use, supraglottic device to support the airway and is available in 7 sizes (Figure 1.3). It is made from thermoplastic elastomer which is inserted supraglottically to form an anatomical seal with the pharyngo-laryngeal structures without the need for any cuff inflation.

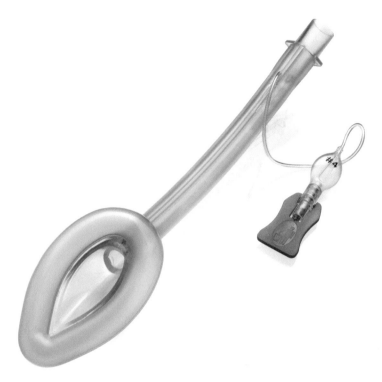

Figure 1.2   Laryngeal Mask Airway. *Courtesy of Intersurgical Ltd.*

What Are the Indications?

These are by and large similar to those for a LMA. The added benefits of i-gels are the rapidity and ease of use, the ability to provide high seal pressures with a conformed anatomical fit, reduced trauma and also a routine gastric port for nasogastric tube insertion to reduce the risk of aspiration. It can serve as a conduit for intubation and as a rescue device in case of a difficult airway.

What Are the Contraindications?

These include trismus, limited mouth opening as well as airway trauma, abscess or mass. Others include obstruction below the glottis and conscious or semi-conscious patients with an intact gag reflex.

Do You Know of Any Other Types of i-gel?

Yes. There is a newer version called i-gel O2.

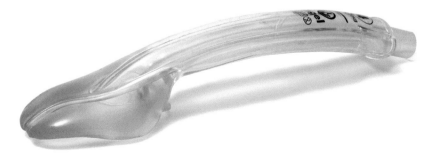

Figure 1.3   i-gel. *Courtesy of Intersurgical Ltd.*

Laryngoscope

What Is This?

This is a Macintosh laryngoscope which is inserted into the mouth to directly visualise the larynx to aid intubation (Figures 1.4 and 1.5). It should be inserted from the right-hand side and advanced into the larynx whilst displacing the tongue to the left.

What Are the Indications?

Its uses include airway management (intubation) when anaesthetising patients and during emergency situations such as cardiac/respiratory arrest when a definitive airway is needed.

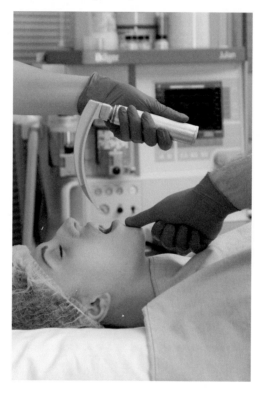

Figure 1.4   Laryngoscope. *Courtesy of Intersurgical Ltd.*

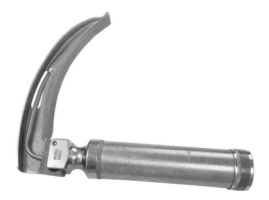

Figure 1.5   Laryngoscope.

What Are the Contraindications?

All contraindications to direct laryngoscopy are relative. Elective intubations should be planned ahead especially if any difficulty is anticipated. Potential difficult intubations may result from limited mouth opening, unstable cervical spine, distorted anatomy from congenital or acquired causes such as radiotherapy and airway obstruction.

Do You Know of Any Complications?

More common complications include trauma to the oral cavity and oropharynx including the teeth. Caution should be undertaken in the presence of loose teeth as they may dislodge and obstruct the airway. Failure to visualise the glottis would warrant further means to facilitate intubation such as a bougie, stylet, video-assisted laryngoscopy and fibreoptic assistance.

Yankauer Suction Tip

What Is This?

This is a Yankauer suction tip which is an oral suctioning device (Figure 1.6). It is a single-use, sterile device. It can be available with or without a control vent. It was developed in the 1900s by an American otolaryngologist, Sidney Yankauer.

What Are the Indications?

It can be used for suctioning oropharyngeal secretions during rapid sequence inductions to prevent aspiration and to ensure a good view of the glottis for intubation. It can also be used in surgical procedures for suctioning of blood and bodily fluids.

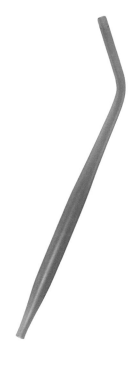

Figure 1.6   Yankauer Suction Tip.

What Are the Contraindications?

It should be used for oral secretions during airway management as inserting it through the nostrils may cause trauma.

Do You Know of Any Complications of Using This Device?

It may cause traumatic tissue grab if not used properly. The suction system should always be checked before initiating a rapid sequence induction to prevent failure of suction.

Oropharyngeal Airway (Guedel)

What Is This?

This is an oropharyngeal (Guedel) airway designed by an American anaesthetist called Arthur Guedel (Figure 1.7). The correct size is chosen by measuring the distance between the patient's mid-point of the maxillary central incisors and the angle of the jaw. In an adult, it is inserted into the mouth upside down displacing the tongue using the curvature and is rotated 180 degrees on contact with the soft palate. It is then advanced further until the flange is in contact with the lips. In children, it is inserted in the correct way up to avoid damage to the soft tissues.

What Are the Indications?

It is usually indicated in unconscious patients to maintain airway patency and to facilitate bag-mask ventilation. It also allows the passage of other devices such as suction catheters and bronchoscopes into the trachea.

What Are the Contraindications?

It should only ever be used in unconscious patients as it may stimulate the gag reflex and induce vomiting leading to an obstructed airway. It should also be avoided in patients with abnormal facial or oropharyngeal anatomy, oral trauma, loose teeth and any foreign body in the upper airway as it may advance the obstruction.

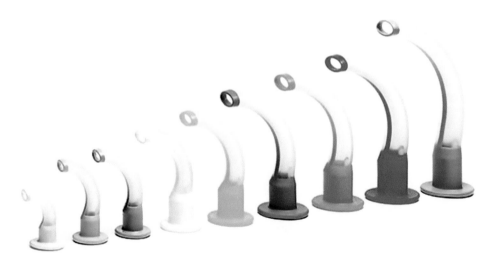

Figure 1.7   Oropharyngeal Airway. *Courtesy of Intersurgical Ltd.*

Do You Know of Any Complications?

Inappropriate use may cause trauma to the lips, teeth and oropharyngeal structures. It may also cause posterior tongue displacement leading to obstruction of the airway.

Nasopharyngeal Airway

What Is This?

This is a nasopharyngeal airway (NPA) (Figure 1.8). It is an uncuffed tube that is inserted nasally reaching beyond the base of the tongue to maintain a patent airway. The correct size is chosen by measuring the distance between the patient's nostril to the angle of the jaw. The airway is lubricated and inserted into the nose until the flange rests on the nostril. A safety pin may be used to prevent advancement of the airway.

What Are the Indications?

It is indicated when airway patency is needed in an unconscious or semiconscious patient through displacement of the tongue and the relaxed upper airway muscles/tissues. It facilitates bag-mask ventilation and allows access of suctioning catheters with minimal trauma to the nasopharyngeal structures. It may also be used in patients in seizures when a patent airway and adequate oxygenation are needed in the short term.

It has the advantage over the Guedel airway in that it can be used in semi-conscious patients as it is better tolerated. It is more ideal than an oropharyngeal airway in the case of locked jaws either due to trismus or iatrogenic causes from maxillofacial surgery.

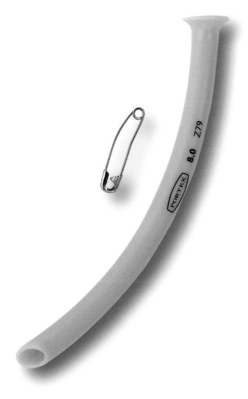

Figure 1.8   Nasopharyngeal Airway. *Courtesy of Smiths Medical.*

What Are the Contraindications?

The absolute contraindications include head and facial trauma where the possibility of a basal skull fracture cannot be ruled out as the NPA could directly penetrate the brain, tear the dura and cause CNS infections. It should be avoided in patients who have undergone trans-sphenoidal surgery and recent rhinoplasty/septoplasty to avoid further trauma.

It should also be avoided in patients with coagulopathy and those on anticoagulation as it may cause severe epistaxis and even profound haemorrhage.

Do You Know of Any Complications?

Inappropriate use may cause damage to the nasopharyngeal structures. Use in contraindicated patients may cause direct damage to the brain and surrounding structures which could lead to severe morbidity and mortality.

Heat and Moisture Exchanger

What Is This?

This is a heat and moisture exchanger (Figure 1.9). It is used in an airway circuit to retain heat and moisture during respiration when the human nose is bypassed. It retains humidification to maintain ciliary action and mucus flow in order to prevent drying of mucus and airway obstruction.

What Are the Indications?

They are generally used in a breathing circuit where the normal function of the human nose to maintain humidification is bypassed. These include any artificial circuits such as those using a laryngeal mask airway, an endotracheal tube or even a tracheostomy.

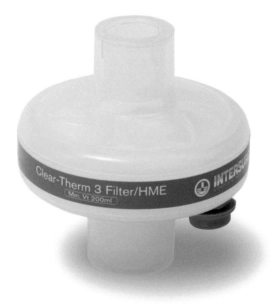

Figure 1.9   Heat and Moisture Exchanger. *Courtesy of Intersurgical Ltd.*

What Are the Contraindications?

These are relative. They may provide inadequate humidification for prolonged use such as those in intensive therapy units. They are also inadequate in warming in hyperventilated patients. In these situations, active heater humidifiers would be more suitable.

What Are the Complications?

It adds further connecting points to the breathing circuit and may risk disconnection. It creates dead space and a small increase in resistance to the gas flow. Obstruction of the circuit may also occur from the patient's respiratory secretions. As a guide, it should be changed every 24 hours.

Tracheostomy Set

What Is This?

This is a tracheostomy set (Figure 1.10). A tracheotomy involves a surgical incision in the trachea to create a passage between the trachea and the skin surface for ventilation. There are two ways of creating a tracheostomy: surgical and percutaneous.

What Are the Indications?

These can be divided into emergency and elective purposes.

Emergency: Upper airway obstruction. This is relatively uncommon nowadays given the advances in tracheal intubation and cricothyroidotomy. However, in cases such as facial injuries, trauma and burns causing swelling or obstruction caused by a foreign object where oral/nasal intubation is not possible and cricothyroidotomy fails, tracheostomy may be required as an emergency airway.

Elective: The most common indication is prolonged ventilation. This reduces dead space in an endotracheal tube and provides easier access and care. It also makes weaning off the ventilator easier. Another indication is the provision of a tracheobronchial toilet.

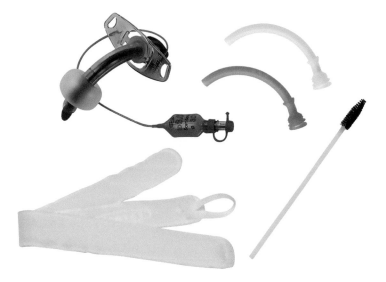

Figure 1.10   Tracheostomy. *Courtesy of Smiths Medical.*

What Are the Contraindications?

There are no absolute contraindications. Relative contraindications include coagulopathy, local infection and cardiovascular/respiratory instability. Another relative contraindication is laryngeal cancer where tracheostomy may prolong the patient's life at the expense of an overgrowing tumour that could further affect cosmesis and quality of life leading to added distress.

What Are the Complications?

These can be divided into immediate, early and late.

Immediate: failure of the procedure leading to respiratory arrest and death, damage to the nearby structures such as the cricoid cartilage, recurrent laryngeal nerve and trachea, bleeding, air embolism, pneumothorax and pain.

Early: Infection, displacement of the tracheostomy, obstruction, pain, swelling, difficulty breathing and subcutaneous emphysema.

Late: scarring, tracheal/subglottic stenosis, tracheo-oesophageal/tracheo-cutaneous/tracheo innominate fistulas, infection, blockage, bacterial colonisation and decannulation.

Intubation Fibrescope

What Is This?

This is an intubation fibrescope (Figure 1.11). It is a long, flexible tube used to facilitate endotracheal intubation nasally or orally. It has a light source attached, a deflectable tip, an instrument channel and an eyepiece at the proximal end. Depending on the model, there can be a charge-coupled device camera attached to the distal or proximal end which can project images onto a screen.

What Are the Indications?

It is used for potentially difficult intubations. Difficult airways are anticipated in patients who have undergone extensive head and neck surgery, certain congenital conditions such as Golderhar syndrome, patients with a high biomedical index (BMI) as well as limited mouth and neck movement. This procedure may be done as an awake intubation with the patient under sedation and topical/local anaesthetic or after the induction of general anaesthetics depending on the risks.

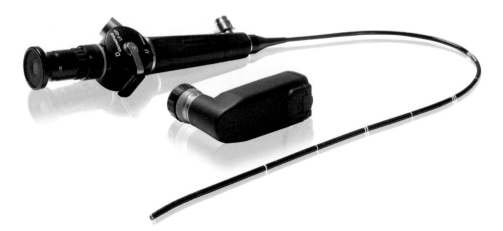

Figure 1.11   Intubation Fibrescope. *Copyright by Olympus Europa SE & Co. KG.*

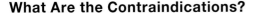

What Are the Contraindications?

Patient refusal and uncooperative patient. Patients with severe maxillofacial trauma or basal skull fractures should not have the procedure done. Excessive bleeding in the airway may render the procedure impossible and dangerous.

What Are the Complications?

These are divided into immediate, early and late.

Immediate: Trauma to the airway, epistaxis, arytenoid/laryngeal injury, pharyngeal haematoma, vocal cord trauma, aspiration and procedural failure leading to death.

Early: Aspiration pneumonia, voice hoarseness and sore throat.

Late: These are rare and are likely due to prolonged intubation. They include: Laryngeal stenosis and tracheal stenosis.

Further Reading

1. Afzal A, Collazo R, Fenves AZ, Schwartz J. Methemoglobinemia precipitated by benzocaine used during intubation. *Proc (Bayl Univ Med Cent)*. 2014;27(2):133–5. PubMed PMID: 24688201; PubMed Central PMCID: PMC3954671.
2. Bonanno FG. The critical airway in adults: The facts. *J Emerg Trauma Shock*. 2012;5(2):153–9. doi: 10.4103/0974-2700.96485. PubMed PMID: 22787346; PubMed Central PMCID: PMC3391840.
3. Kim HJ, Kim SH, Min NH, Park WK. Determination of the appropriate sizes of oropharyngeal airways in adults: Correlation with external facial measurements: A randomised crossover study. *Eur J Anaesthesiol*. 2016;33(12):936–942. PubMed PMID: 26908003.
4. Roberts K, Whalley H, Bleetman A. The nasopharyngeal airway: Dispelling myths and establishing the facts. *Emerg Med J*. 2005;22(6):394–6. Review. PubMed PMID: 15911941; PubMed Central PMCID: PMC1726817.

BREATHING

1) Nasal Cannula
2) Venturi Mask
3) Non-Rebreathe Mask

Nasal Cannula

What Are These?

These are nasal cannulae (Figure 2.1). They provide oxygen at an inspiratory oxygen fraction (FiO$_2$) of 24–40 % (1–5 L/min) through the nose. The actual flow rate is affected by the respiratory rate and tidal volumes.

What Are the Indications?

It is indicated in patients requiring low oxygen support. It is often used with 2L O$_2$/min giving 24% of O$_2$. These include people with O$_2$ demand due to atelectasis, pneumonia and during recovery post-operatively.

What Are the Contraindications?

Care should be taken in patients at risk of CO$_2$ retention.

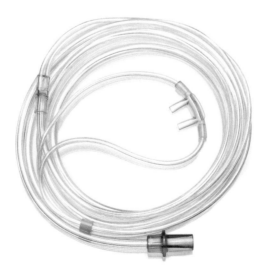

Figure 2.1   Nasal Cannula. *Courtesy of Intersurgical Ltd.*

What Are the Complications?

CO_2 retention is a potential complication. Any flow rate over 2 L could cause discomfort and drying of nasal mucosa.

Venturi Masks

What Is This?

These are Venturi masks (Figures 2.2 through 2.6). It provides oxygen at different concentrations according to different flow rate settings. It provides accurate and constant oxygen flow concentrations at 24%, 28%, 31%, 35%, 40%, 50% and 60%; the respective colours are blue, white, orange, yellow, red, pink and green.

What Are the Indications?

It is indicated in patients requiring oxygen supplementation where accurate titration is desired. These include pneumonia, atelectasis and pneumothorax. It is often employed in patients where CO_2 retention is a concern.

What Are the Contraindications?

Titration is needed when there is a risk of CO_2 retention.

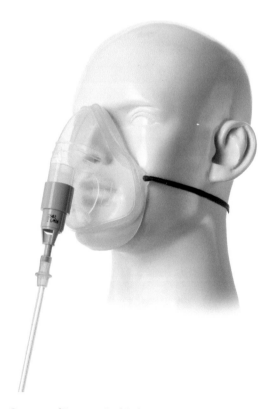

Figure 2.2   Venturi Mask. *Courtesy of Intersurgical Ltd.*

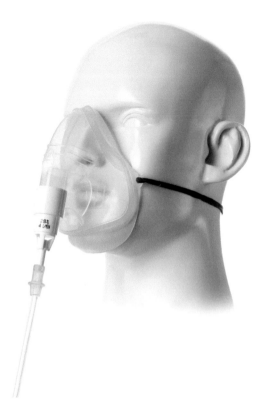

Figure 2.3   Venturi Mask. *Courtesy of Intersurgical Ltd.*

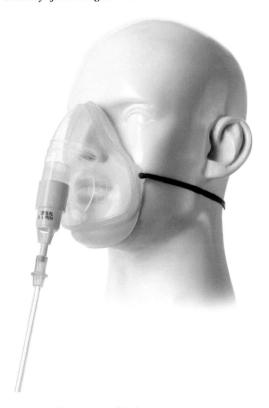

Figure 2.4   Venturi Mask. *Courtesy of Intersurgical Ltd.*

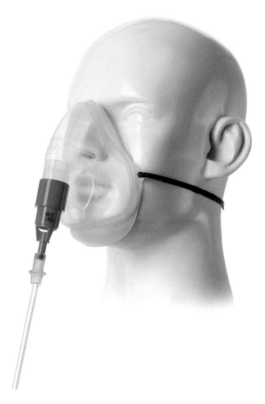

Figure 2.5 Venturi Mask. *Courtesy of Intersurgical Ltd.*

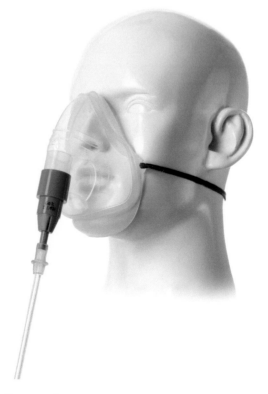

Figure 2.6 Venturi Mask. *Courtesy of Intersurgical Ltd.*

What Are the Complications?

CO_2 retention in patients requiring a hypoxic respiratory drive.

Non-Rebreathe Mask

What Is This?

This is a non-rebreathe mask (Figure 2.7). It has a reservoir bag and a one-way valve to deliver high flow oxygen. The reservoir bag is filled with oxygen so long as the patient's rate of breathing is less than that of the O2 flow. The patient then preferentially breathes in from the reservoir bag ensuring minimal mixture with ambient air.

What Are the Indications?

It is indicated when the patient has a high oxygen demand (i.e. >40% FiO2). These include any emergency situation of desaturation, pulmonary embolism and pneumothorax. It can theoretically deliver up to 90% of O2 if used correctly.

What Are the Contraindications?

CO_2 retention should be a concern for people at risk such as patients suffering from COPD.

What Are the Complications?

Care should always be taken to ensure that the reservoir bag is filled before use so that maximum O_2 can be delivered for the intended use. CO2 retention may be a potential complication.

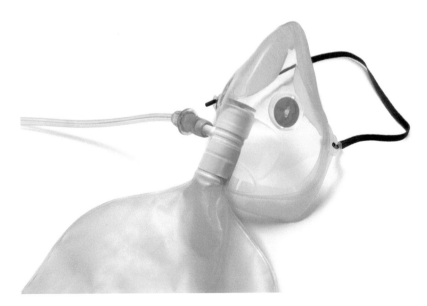

Figure 2.7   Non-Rebreathe Mask. *Courtesy of Intersurgical Ltd.*

CIRCULATION

1) Intravenous Cannula
2) Arterial Catheter
3) Central Venous Catheter
4) Peripherally Inserted Central Catheter
5) Skin-Tunnelled Central Venous Catheter
6) Skin-Tunnelled Dialysis Catheter
7) Plasma-Lyte 148
8) Hartmann's Solution
9) Normal Saline
10) Swan–Ganz Catheter
11) Automated External Defibrillator

Intravenous Cannula

What Is This?

This is an intravenous cannula (Figure 3.1). As its name suggests, it is inserted into the vein to provide peripheral intravenous access. They come in different sizes at 26 G, 24 G, 22 G, 20 G, 18 G,

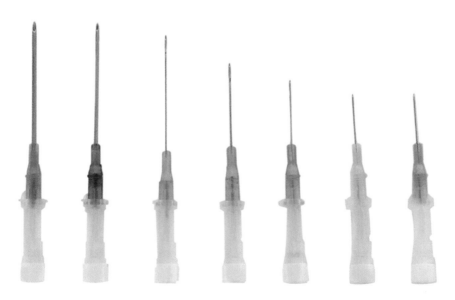

Figure 3.1 Intravenous Cannulas. *Courtesy of Smiths Medical.*

16 G and 14 G and are colour-coded ranging from violet, yellow, blue, pink, green, grey and orange at increasing sizes respectively. As the maximum flow rate through a cannula is proportional to its diameter, the smaller the gauge the higher the flow rate:

Gauge	Colour	Flow Rate ml/min
14 G	Orange	240
16 G	Grey	180
18 G	Green	90
20 G	Pink	60
22 G	Blue	36
24 G	Yellow	20
26 G	Violet	10–15

What Are the Indications?

The main indications are for IV medications and fluids. It is particularly important in an emergency situation (e.g. cardiac arrest, shock) when resuscitation drugs and fluids such as inotropes, vasopressors and blood products are needed. The flow rate is of particular importance in this setting especially in patients in shock where a high volume of fluid has to be infused within a short timeframe.

What Are the Contraindications?

These are relative. They should be avoided in sites of infection, burns and injury.

What Are the Complications?

The most common ones include pain, ecchymosis, double punctures and "tissued" cannulas. Less common complications include nerve damage, arterial puncture, thrombophlebitis and tissue necrosis. As a guide, it should be changed every 72 hours.

Arterial Catheter

What Is This?

These are arterial catheters (Figures 3.2 through 3.4). It is inserted into an artery either by simple cannulation or by the Seldinger technique. It is then connected to a transducer which converts kinetic energy from the pulse waves to electrical energy which is displayed onto a computer screen. It is also connected to a bag of fluid with a fixed flow rate to keep the line patent.

What Are the Indications?

These include continuous monitoring of blood pressure, frequent blood sampling and blood gas sampling.

What Are the Contraindications?

An arterial line should not be inserted where there is a risk of compromising distal circulation. Such cases include Buerger's Disease, Raynaud's syndrome and end arteries such as the brachial

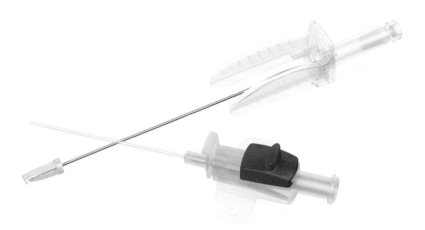

Figure 3.2   Arterial Catheter. *Courtesy of Vygon (UK) Ltd.*

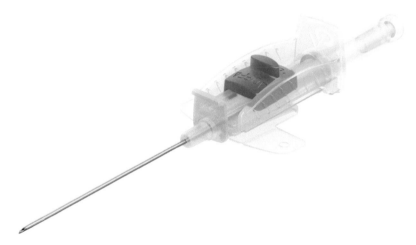

Figure 3.3   Arterial Catheter. *Courtesy of Vygon (UK) Ltd.*

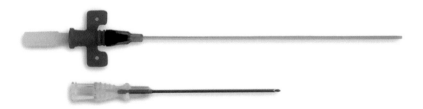

Figure 3.4   Arterial Catheter. *Courtesy of Vygon (UK) Ltd.*

artery. Other contraindications include a present infection at the site of insertion, presence of an AV shunt and burns over the cannulation site.

Do You Know of Any Test That May Help to Determine Whether an Artery Is Suitable For an Arterial Line?

Yes – Allen's test. It involves occluding the radial and ulnar arteries sequentially to identify the adequacy of collaterals in the case of a radial arterial line.

What Are the Complications?

Common complications include bleeding and haematoma. Less common complications include infection, thrombosis, ischaemic damage distal to the cannulation site, nerve injury and pseudoaneurysm.

Central Venous Catheter

What Is This?

This is a central venous catheter which is inserted into a central vein such as the internal jugular, subclavian and femoral veins (Figure 3.5). It is inserted using the Seldinger technique under ultrasound guidance. A central vein is first identified by its compressibility, a needle attached to a syringe is then inserted with negative pressure applied until blood is aspirated, a guidewire is then advanced through the needle followed by dilatation of the skin and subcutaneous tissues before the central venous catheter is inserted. A CXR is usually performed to confirm the position of the line. A blood gas analysis can also be done to confirm the venous placement of the catheter. It is usually a triple-lumen catheter where different ports are used for medication administration, IV fluids and the measurement of central venous pressure.

What Are the Indications?

These can be divided into investigative and therapeutic purposes. For investigation, it can be used for measuring the central venous pressure to estimate the preload and blood volume of the patient or the central venous oxygenation for the purpose of goal-directed therapy. For treatment, it is used to administer drugs such as chemotherapy agents and vasopressors that are irritant to peripheral veins. Total parental nutrition is also delivered via a central line due to its concentrated content and the subsequent risk of thrombosis. It is often used when peripheral IV access is difficult and that immediate venous access is needed.

What Are the Contraindications?

These include infection at the insertion site and known anatomical anomalies such as arterio-venous malformations and known vascular injuries/previous surgery. An absolute contraindication

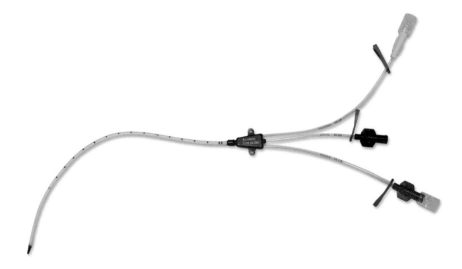

Figure 3.5   Central Venous Catheter. *Courtesy of Smiths Medical.*

for a subclavian approach is coagulopathy where compression is not possible in case of bleeding. Other contraindications include burned sites and uncooperative patients.

Do You Know of Any Complications?

Immediate complications include failure of the procedure, arterial cannulation/puncture, bleeding, pneumothorax, haemothorax, air embolism, haematoma and arrhythmia.

Early complications include infection and a blocked catheter.

Late complications include infection, thrombosis, vascular stenosis and erosion.

In removing the catheter, the patient should be tilted head-down and the catheter pulled out whilst performing the Valsalva manoeuvre in order to minimise the risk of air embolism.

Peripherally Inserted Central Catheter

What Is This?

This is a peripherally inserted central catheter (PICC) (Figure 3.6). It is inserted peripherally such as in the brachial, basilic or cephalic veins. It is safer to insert than central lines and is easier to manage in the community in the long term (up to 6 months).

What Are the Indications?

PICC is indicated in patients when regular IV therapy is required for up to 6 months. These include parental nutrition, long-term antibiotics and chemotherapy. This is particularly true when the IV drug used is an irritant.

What Are the Contraindications?

PICC is indicated for IV access in the medium term (up to 6 months). If long-term IV access is required, PICC should not be used.

What Are the Complications?

There can be divided into immediate, early and late.

Immediate: Damage to nearby structures, pain, air embolism and cardiac arrhythmia.

Early: Thrombosis, infection, malposition, thrombophlebitis and haematoma.

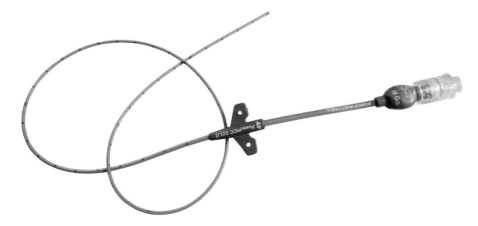

Figure 3.6   Peripherally Inserted Central Catheter. *Courtesy of Dr Richard Leech, Kent Vascular Access.*

Late: Infection, thrombosis, fracture of catheter and the resultant embolisation and malposition.

Point of note – Although a PICC can be a convenient alternative to lines such as the Hickman and can be inserted by nursing staff on the ward, the catheter tip is difficult to manipulate. Malposition occurs in 25–40% of the cases. Thrombosis occurs in 21% of cases but rises rapidly to up to 60% if the tip sits in any of the axillary, subclavian or innominate vessels (Galloway and Bodenham, 2004; Kearns et al., 1996).

Skin-Tunnelled Central Venous Catheter

What Is This?

This is a skin-tunnelled central venous catheter (Figure 3.7). The most common type is the Hickman line which had an original internal diameter of 1.6 mm. It now comes in various sizes. It is used to provide long-term vascular access (months to years) for blood-taking and the administration of irritant drugs. It aims to reduce the rate of infection by increasing the distance between the skin entry and the blood vessel puncture sites. It is usually inserted by an interventional radiologist as a minor surgical procedure under local anaesthetic. It is commonly inserted through the jugular or the subclavian vein into the superior vena cava under ultrasound or X-ray guidance. The other end of the tip is then tunnelled under the skin which then comes out through an incision made in the chest skin. A Dacron cuff exists around the tube where subcutaneous fibrosis occurs to prevent accidental dislodgement.

What Are the Indications?

Skin-tunnelled catheters are indicated in patients requiring long-term vascular access for regular blood transfusions and irritant/vesicant drugs. It can be used for frequent blood samples whilst avoiding regular venepunctures. Total parenteral nutrition can also be given via this route.

What Are the Contraindications?

Neutropaenia, thrombocytopaenia and clotting factor abnormalities would generally contraindicate the procedure. Patients with any active infection should not have the procedure done.

What Are the Complications?

These can be divided into immediate, early and late. However, the most common complications are infection and thrombotic occlusion.

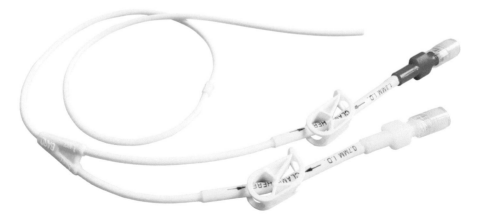

Figure 3.7   Skin-Tunnelled Central Venous Catheter. *Courtesy of Dr Richard Leech, Kent Vascular Access.*

Immediate: Pneumothorax, haemothorax, damage to nearby structures/blood vessels and pain.

Early: Thrombosis, local haematoma, pain and infection.

Late: Catheter malfunction such as drug extravasation, catheter damage/fracture and the resultant embolisation/thrombosis, and infection.

Skin-Tunnelled Dialysis Catheter

What Is This?

This is a Tesio line which is a skin-tunnelled central venous catheter used for dialysis and apheresis (Figure 3.8). It consists of 2 separate tubes to provide de facto double-lumen access. It is usually inserted into the internal jugular vein until the tip reaches the superior vena cava. It is generally used as a medium-term catheter for up to 6 months but can be used for longer if needed. The Tesio line has two single lumina with an internal diameter of 2 mm each and provides a mean flow rate in excess of 300 ml/min making it ideal for dialysis.

What Are the Indications?

It is mainly used as a temporary measure for dialysis when an arteriovenous fistula is not available. Less commonly, it can be used in patients who need regular red cell exchange and apheresis.

What Are the Contraindications?

Active infection is an absolute contraindication. Neutropenia, thrombocytopenia and clotting factor abnormalities would generally contraindicate the procedure.

What Are the Complications?

These can be divided into immediate, early and late. However, more common complications are infection and thrombotic occlusion.

Immediate: Pneumothorax, haemothorax, damage to nearby structures and blood vessels, and pain.

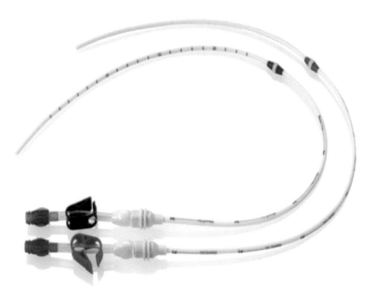

Figure 3.8   Skin-Tunnelled Dialysis Catheter. *Courtesy of Utano Africa.*

Early: Thrombosis, local haematoma, pain and infection.

Late: Catheter malfunction such as drug extravasation, catheter damage and fracture and the resultant embolisation/thrombosis, and infection.

Plasma-Lyte 148

What Is This?

This is a balanced isotonic crystalloid solution with electrolytes, pH and osmolality that closely mimic human plasma (Figure 3.9). It is a buffered solution containing acetate and gluconate.

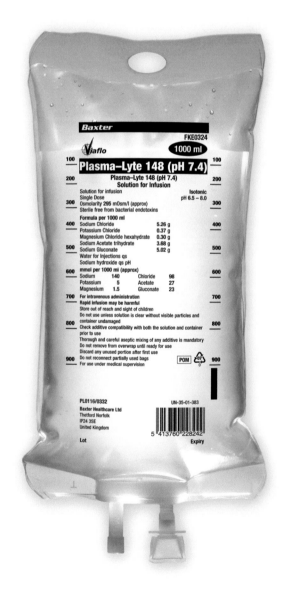

Figure 3.9   Plasma-Lyte 148. *Courtesy of Baxter.*

A typical 1L bag of Plasma-Lyte 148 contains the following:

pH	7.4
Osmolarity	295 mOsm/l (approx.)
Na$^+$	140 mmol/l
K$^+$	5.0 mmol/l
Mg $^{++}$	1.5 mmol/l
Cl$^-$	98 mmol/l
Acetate$^-$	27 mmol/l
Gluconate	23 mmol/l

What Are the Indications?

The main indication is fluid replacement. This may be in the cases of burns, infection, during pre-operative fast, intraoperative fluid loss and dehydration. Other indications include resuscitative situations such as hypovolaemic and septic shocks. Plasma-Lyte is also indicated in mild to moderate metabolic acidosis and in cases of lactate metabolism impairment.

What Are the Contraindications?

It is an absolute contraindication in patients with hypersensitivity to the contents of Plasma-Lyte. Given the relatively high potassium content, patients with hyperkalaemia and renal failure should not be given Plasma-Lyte. IV fluid therapy should always be used cautiously especially in patients with heart failure, renal failure and pulmonary oedema.

What Are the Complications?

As it comes in a flexible plastic bag, connecting it with other bags of fluids in a series or not emptying residual air in the bag before connection can result in air embolism.

Depending on patient characteristics and the volume/rate of administration, it can cause fluid overload leading to pulmonary oedema, electrolyte disturbances and acid-base imbalance.

Hartmann's Solution

What Is This?

This is called Hartmann's solution which is a balanced isotonic crystalloid solution (Figure 3.10). It is a buffered solution containing lactate.

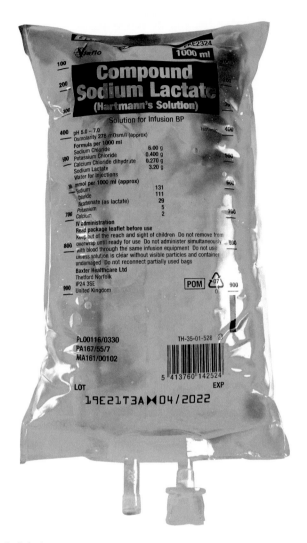

Figure 3.10   Hartmann's Solution.

A typical 1L bag of Hartmann's solution contains the following:

pH	5.0-7.0
Osmolarity	278 mOsm/l (approx.)
Na+	131 mmol/l
K+	5.0 mmol/l
Cl-	111 mmol/l
Ca++	2 mmol/l
Lactate (Bicarbonate)	29 mmol/l

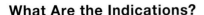

What Are the Indications?

The most common indication is fluid replacement. This may be in the cases of burns, infection, during pre-operative fast, intraoperative fluid loss and dehydration. Hartmann's solution is also indicated in mild to moderate metabolic acidosis except for lactic acidosis.

What Are the Contraindications?

Patients with known hypersensitivity to any of the contents should not be given Hartmann's. Concomitant administration of ceftriaxone with Hartmann's is contraindicated because of the risk of precipitation. It should be given cautiously in patients with congestive heart failure or severe renal impairment requiring haemodialysis depending on the indication, as fluid overload is common. It should also be used cautiously in hyperkalaemic patients. It is not used to treat lactic acidosis. Lactate can be converted to glucose via the Cori cycle and should be used cautiously in diabetic patients. It should be used very cautiously in patients on digitalis therapy due to the risk of calcium-enhanced drug effects and drugs that increase the vasopressin effect owing to the risk of hyponatraemia.

What Are the Complications?

More common complications include fluid overload, electrolyte imbalance and administration errors including air embolism.

Normal Saline

What Is This?

This is a 0.9% sodium chloride intravenous infusion solution (Figure 3.11). It is a crystalloid solution.

A typical 1L bag of Normal Saline contains the following:

pH	5.5 (Approx.)
Osmolarity	308 mOsm/l
Na^+	154 mmol/l
Cl^-	154 mmol/l

What Are the Indications?

The main indication is fluid replacement for isotonic extracellular dehydration. It can also be used to treat hyponatraemia. It is commonly used as a vehicle for compatible drugs in parenteral administration.

What Are the Contraindications?

It is contraindicated in patients with hypernatraemia and hyperchloraemia. It should be used cautiously in patients with congestive heart failure and renal impairment requiring haemodialysis due to the risk of fluid overload.

What Are the Complications?

More common complications include fluid overload, hypernatraemia and hyperchloraemia.

Rapidly correcting hyponatraemia can lead to central pontine myelinolysis.

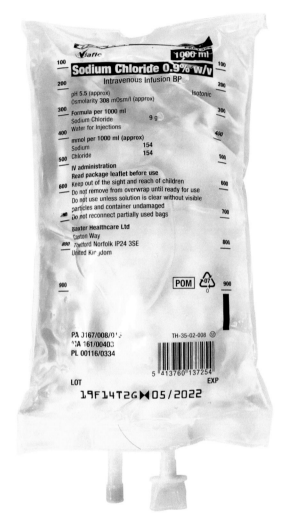

Figure 3.11   Normal Saline.

Swan–Ganz Catheter

What Is This?

This is a pulmonary artery catheter, also called a Swan–Ganz catheter (Figure 3.12). It is a multi-lumen catheter with an inflatable balloon at the tip. It is inserted like a central line into a central vein. However, it further goes into the right atrium, the right ventricle, the pulmonary artery, thence to a pulmonary artery branch where the balloon is inflated in order to calculate the pulmonary capillary wedge pressure.

What Are the Indications?

The main indication is to determine the volume status of the patient. This is usually done by using a central line to measure the central venous pressure (CVP). However, there are scenarios in which the CVP is unreliable in determining volume status as it relies on the correlation with the filling pressures of the atria. These can be affected by disease states such as valvular disease, pulmonary

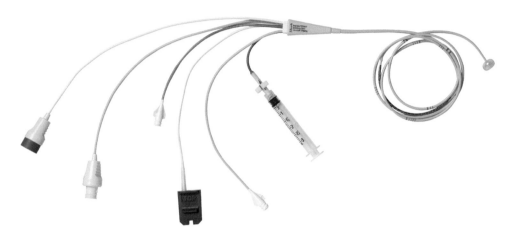

Figure 3.12 Swan–Ganz Catheter. *Swan-Ganz™ pulmonary artery catheter, courtesy of Edwards Lifesciences Corporation.*

oedema from left ventricular failure, interstitial pulmonary oedema and chronic lung disease. In these cases, a pulmonary artery catheter is indicated for the assessment of volume status.

What Are the Contraindications?

Given the course of the insertion of a pulmonary artery catheter, damage to anything along the way may pose risks to insertion. These include prosthetic and vegetated tricuspid and pulmonary valves as well as tumour/thrombus within the right heart or the vessels involved. Active endocarditis would contraindicate the procedure.

What Are the Complications?

These can be classified as immediate, early and late.

Immediate: Pneumothorax, haemothorax, damage to the SVC, valves, endocardium and myocardium, atrial and ventricular arrhythmia, pulmonary infarction, air embolism and pulmonary artery rupture.

Early: Thromboembolism, endocarditis and infection.

Late: Scarring and arteriovenous fistula.

Automated External Defibrillator

What Is This?

This is an automated external defibrillator (AED) (Figure 3.13). It is an electrical device that discharges pre-programmed levels of energy across the myocardium to depolarise myocardial cells synchronously to achieve a sinus rhythm. It has a capacitor which stores electrical energy before discharge on command. Most AEDs have the function to provide synchronised electrical shocks for cardioversion. This can be used to treat arrhythmia in patients electively or emergently.

What Are the Indications?

Defibrillation is the only effective treatment for ventricular fibrillation. An automated external defibrillator allows the restoration of sinus rhythm through breaking the cycle of uncoordinated ventricular depolarisations thereby allowing the sinus atrial node to re-establish the sinus rhythm through coordinated depolarisations. It is also used to treat pulseless ventricular tachycardia.

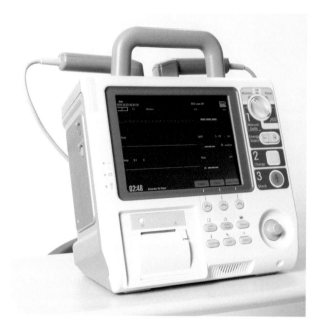

Figure 3.13   Automated External Defibrillator.

The synchronised function is used to treat supraventricular tachycardia in patients who are haemodynamically unstable but still have a pulse in an emergency situation. It can also be used to electively treat atrial fibrillation (AF) where sedation should be given. This may be accompanied by anticoagulation beforehand depending on the time of onset of the AF. The recommended energy levels for this purpose range from 50 to 200 joules.

What Are the Contraindications?

Defibrillation – if the patient is conscious and responsive, defibrillation should never be given.

Synchronised cardioversion – there is no absolute contraindication to this except for patient refusal. Implanted cardiac devices do not affect the indication of the procedure.

What Are the Complications?

These can be divided into patient and bystander harm.

Patient harm: Delivering an electrical shock to a patient with a sinus rhythm can cause a cardiac arrest. Failure to deliver an electrical shock due to device failure or human error may result in death. Myocardial damage, skin burns and skin allergies to the pads of the AED may also happen.

Bystander harm: Fire hazard especially in the close proximity of high oxygen concentration and flammable gases. Shocks could be accidentally delivered to resuscitators and bystanders if not properly used.

Further Reading

1. Atherikul K, Schwab SJ, Conlon PJ. Adequacy of haemodialysis with cuffed central-vein catheters. *Nephrol Dial Transplant.* 1998;13(3):745–9. PubMed PMID: 9550658.

2. Cheung E, Baerlocher MO, Asch M, Myers A. Venous access: A practical review for 2009. *Can Fam Physician*. 2009;55(5):494–6. Review. PubMed PMID: 19439704; PubMed Central PMCID: PMC2682308.

3. Galloway S, Bodenham A. Long-term central venous access. *Br J Anaesth*. 2004;92(5):722–34. Epub 2004 Mar 5. Review. PubMed PMID: 15003979.

4. Goerig M, Agarwal K, Schulte am Esch J. The versatile August Bier (1861–1949), father of spinal anesthesia. *J Clin Anesth*. 2000;12(7):561–9. PubMed PMID: 11137420.

5. Goyal A, Sciammarella JC, Chhabra L, Singhal M. Synchronized electrical cardioversion. 2019 July 4. StatPearls [Internet]. Treasure Island, FL: StatPearls Publishing; 2019 Jan. Available from http://www.ncbi.nlm.nih.gov/books/NBK482173/. PubMed PMID: 29489237.

6. Kearns PJ, Coleman S, Wehner JH. Complications of long arm-catheters: A randomized trial of central vs peripheral tip location. *JPEN J Parenter Enteral Nutr*. 1996;20(1):20–4. PubMed PMID: 8788259.

7. Kornbau C, Lee KC, Hughes GD, Firstenberg MS. Central line complications. *Int J Crit Illn Inj Sci*. 2015;5(3):170–8. doi: 10.4103/2229-5151.164940. PubMed PMID: 26557487; PubMed Central PMCID: PMC4613416.

8. Weisz Michael T. Physical principles of defibrillators. *Anaest Intens Care Med*. 2009;10(8):367–369. ISSN 1472-0299, doi: 10.1016/j.mpaic.2009.05.002.

9. Trerotola SO, Kraus M, Shah H, Namyslowski J, Johnson MS, Stecker MS, Ahmad I, McLennan G, Patel NH, O'Brien E, Lane KA, Ambrosius WT. Randomized comparison of split tip versus step tip high-flow hemodialysis catheters. *Kidney Int*. 2002;62(1):282–9. PubMed PMID: 12081590.

ANALGESIA

4

1) Spinal Needle
2) Epidural Set
3) Patient-controlled Analgesia Machine

Spinal Needle

What Is This?

These are spinal needles (Figures 4.1 and 4.2). It is inserted into the subarachnoid space at the lower lumbar level in order to provide a spinal anaesthetic. The layers of penetration of the spinal needle are the skin, subcutaneous fat, supraspinous ligament, interspinous ligament, ligamentum flavum, dura mater and arachnoid mater. The first spinal anaesthetic was performed by August Bier in 1898. The Whitacre needle features a pencil point tip which is thought to minimise the risk of post-puncture headache. The Quincke needle has a bevelled tip which cuts parallel to the dura fibres.

What Are the Indications?

Surgery in the lower body including Caesarean section and lower limb procedures. Spinal anaesthetic has the added benefit of post-operative analgesia depending on the duration of the procedure and the dose/type of anaesthetic used.

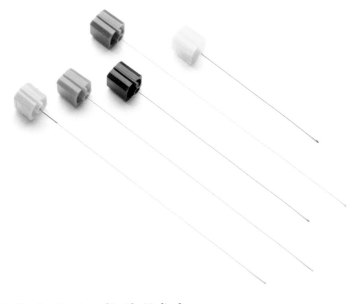

Figure 4.1 Quincke Needle. *Courtesy of Smiths Medical.*

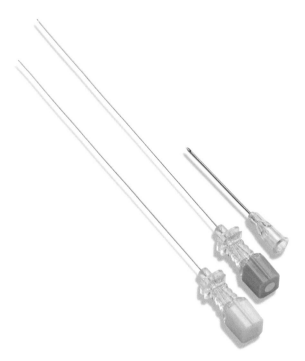

Figure 4.2   Whitacre needle. *Courtesy of Smiths Medical.*

What Are the Contraindications?

Absolute contraindications include warfarinised patients, patients who have not stopped taking clopidogrel for at least 5 days before the procedure, coagulopathy, infection at the site of puncture, severe aortic stenosis and patient refusal. Relative contraindications include uncooperative patients and pre-existing neurological deficits.

What Are the Complications?

Post-procedural headaches and hypotension are fairly common side effects. The rest are uncommon but include bleeding, infection and neurological damage. There is also a risk of procedure failure which would dictate the conversion to a general anaesthetic should the procedure go ahead.

Epidural Set

What Is This?

This is an epidural set (Figure 4.3). It consists of an epidural needle, a catheter and a loss of resistance syringe. It is inserted at any level along the spinal cord into the epidural space using the loss of resistance (LOR) technique to provide both anaesthesia and analgesia for surgery and analgesia in labour.

What Are the Indications?

It is commonly used for analgesia in labour and other abdominal surgery both intraoperatively and postoperatively. Other indications include providing anaesthesia for abdominal, pelvic and lower limb surgery. More rarely it may be used as a cervical epidural for procedures such as carotid endarterectomy and hand surgery.

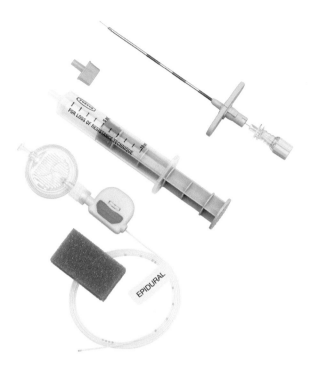

Figure 4.3   Epidural Set. *Courtesy of Smiths Medical.*

What Are the Contraindications?

These are similar to those of a spinal anaesthetic and include infection at the site of cannulation, allergy to the anaesthetic of choice and patient refusal. Other contraindications include coagulopathy, low platelets, current warfarin use and severe stenotic cardiac disease such as aortic stenosis.

Are There Any Complications?

Yes. Common immediate complications include failure of procedure, pain, hypotension and itching (if opioid is used). Common early to late complications include further spread of local anaesthetic affecting the respiratory muscles and the phrenic nerve leading to respiratory depression, sympathetic supply to the heart leading to bradycardia and cranial nerves leading to nerve palsies.

Patient-Controlled Analgesia Machine

What Is This?

This is a patient-controlled analgesia (PCA) machine (Figures 4.4 and 4.5). It is used to deliver analgesic drugs on demand. It has a patient-controlled button which directs the pump to deliver the drug of choice at a set dose when pressed. In most cases, the machine supplies opioid drugs such as morphine and fentanyl. The pump is connected to a tube which is typically attached to the patient intravenously or epidurally. PCA through a peripheral nerve catheter has gained increasing popularity in recent years. More recent studies have also shown the efficacy of PCA through other routes of administration such as transdermal, sublingual, oral and inhalational. All PCA machines should have the functions to deliver a loading dose, boluses on demand, a background infusion as well as lockout intervals and hourly or 4-hourly limits.

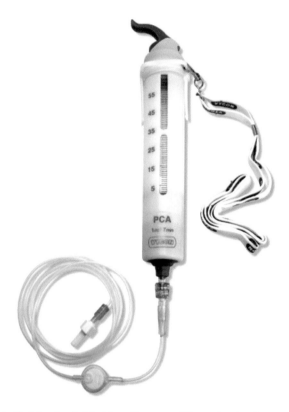

Figure 4.4   Patient-Controlled Analgesia Machine. *Courtesy of Vygon (UK) Ltd.*

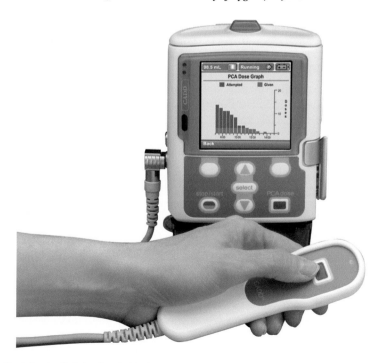

Figure 4.5   Patient-Controlled Analgesia Machine. *Courtesy of Merit Medical UK.*

What Are the Indications?

PCA is used to manage moderate to severe pain for which intermittent oral and IV morphine is inadequate. The most common indication is post-operative pain control. For example, upper gastrointestinal tract surgery typically requires an epidural anaesthetic. The use of an epidural PCA would be indicated in this setting. Abdominal surgery would usually require an intravenous PCA postoperatively. Other indications include severe acute pain, acute exacerbation of chronic pain, cancer pain and pain otherwise uncontrolled by usual routes of administration.

What Are the Contraindications?

Known allergies should preclude the use of certain drugs. Patients with a reduced Glasgow Coma Scale (GCS) or a lack of mental capacity to understand the rationale of the analgesic method should not be given a PCA.

Point of note: PCA usage should be monitored. If the patient is using rescue doses too frequently, the usual oral analgesic regimen and sustained-release form should be adjusted accordingly.

What Are the Complications?

There can be divided into drug and machine issues.

Drugs:

Opioid side effects include sedation, nausea, vomiting, addiction, constipation and respiratory depression.

Local anaesthetic side effects include:

Localised symptoms: motor weakness and paraesthesia

Systemic symptoms: central nervous system toxicity such as confusion, agitation, convulsions, coma and respiratory depression. Cardiovascular system toxicity such as myocardial depression, severe arrhythmias and hypotension.

Machine-related issues: malfunction leading to over- and under-dosing, disconnection, tube kinking and infection.

Further Reading

1. Dickerson DM, Apfelbaum JL. Local anesthetic systemic toxicity. *Aesthet Surg J.* 2014;34(7):1111–9. doi: 10.1177/1090820X14543102. Epub 2014 Jul 15. Review. PubMed PMID: 25028740.
2. Fettes PD, Jansson JR, Wildsmith JA. Failed spinal anaesthesia: Mechanisms, management, and prevention. *Br J Anaesth.* 2009;102(6):739–48. doi: 10.1093/bja/aep096. Epub 2009 May 6. Review. PubMed PMID: 19420004.
3. Mann C, Pouzeratte Y, Boccara G, Peccoux C, Vergne C, Brunat G, Domergue J, Millat B, Colson P. Comparison of intravenous or epidural patient-controlled analgesia in the elderly after major abdominal surgery. *Anesthesiology.* 2000;92(2):433–41. PubMed PMID: 10691230.
4. Wadlund DL. Local anesthetic systemic toxicity. *AORN J.* 2017;106(5):367–377. doi: 10.1016/j.aorn.2017.08.015. PubMed PMID: 29107256.

Part Two

SURGICAL INSTRUMENTS

CARDIOTHORACIC

5

1) Chest Drain Set
2) Trocar
3) Underwater Seal Device

Chest Drain Set

What Is This?

This is a chest drain set (Figure 5.1). It has a selection of syringes and needles, a scalpel, a blade, sutures, a guidewire, a dilator, a chest tube and a closed drainage system. The chest drain is available in different sizes typically ranging from 8 Ch to 36 Ch. It can be inserted by thoracotomy or using the Seldinger technique with a guidewire. Although the British Thoracic Society (BTS) guidelines strongly recommend that this procedure should be done under ultrasound guidance, clear understanding of the anatomical landmarks is important. The preferred site of chest drain insertion is the safety triangle. This is defined as the space bordered superiorly by the base of the axilla, anteriorly by the lateral edge of the pectoralis major, inferiorly by the 5th intercostal space and laterally by the lateral edge of the latissimus dorsi muscle. The needle should be inserted just above a rib to avoid damage to the neurovascular bundle though the lower the rib is, the less likely it is that the rib flange will cover the bundle and as such, a more anterior site may avoid damage

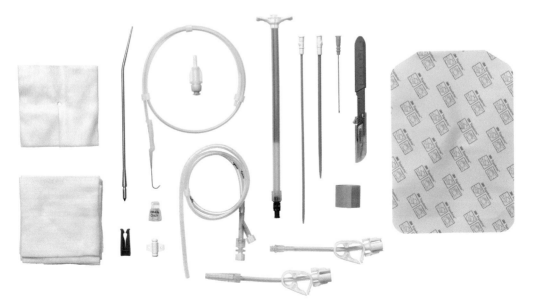

Figure 5.1   Chest Drain Set. *Courtesy of Merit Medical UK.*

(Carney and Ravin, 1979; Havelock et al., 2010). The chest tube is secured at the skin using the sutures provided. The chest drain should be connected to a closed drainage system to prevent entrapping air or fluid into the pleural cavity. A wide range of systems can be used including the underwater seal, flutter valve or a multifunction chest drainage system.

What Are the Indications?

There are several indications for the insertion of a chest drain. These include pneumothorax and pleural effusion. It is, however, important to note that spontaneous pneumothoraces do not necessarily require a chest drain according to the BTS guideline. In certain cases, conservative management with high flow oxygen may be adequate. Ventilated patients or patients likely to undergo ventilation should have a chest drain inserted to prevent further complications of the pneumothorax.

What Are the Contraindications?

As per the BTS guideline, certain spontaneous pneumothoraces do not require a chest drain and can be managed conservatively with high-flow oxygen or simple aspiration. Tension pneumothorax is a medical emergency and should not be managed with a chest drain until the tension is relieved by decompression. This is done by inserting a cannula in the 2nd intercostal space in the mid-clavicular line on the side of the pneumothorax. Patient refusal is also an absolute contraindication. If not an emergency, clotting profile should be checked before the procedure and an INR <1.5 should be aimed.

What Are the Complications, If Any?

These can be divided into immediate, early and late complications. Immediate complications include damage to the nearby anatomical structures. These include injuries to the intercostal blood vessels or other large vessels from which haemorrhage may result. Damage to the nearby organs/structures such as the heart and nerves may be possible. Although local anaesthetic is used, pain is a common feature. Procedural failure such as incorrect placement of the drain can occur.

Early complications include a rapid shift in the pleural pressure if a (usually large) pleural effusion is drained rapidly. This is caused by the rapid re-expansion of the collapsed lung leading to pulmonary oedema. The mortality rate of this has been shown to be as high as 20%. Slow and careful monitoring of drainage is therefore advised. Usually no more than 1.5 L of fluid should be drained per attempt (sometimes per day). The chest drain should be clamped at this point. The patient should be monitored for any symptoms such as shortness of breath, cough, tachycardia, hypotension and pain. If suction is used, an experienced nurse should be present to avoid using a low-volume high-pressure pump or a high-pressure wall suction regulator. If clamping of the drain occurs when there is an air leak, a tension pneumothorax can occur.

Late complications include infection and re-accumulation of pleural fluids/recurrent pneumothorax.

Trocar

What Is This?

This is a trocar used for the insertion of a chest drain (Figure 5.2). It can have a sharp or a blunt end. It has historically been used to create a track into the pleural space to guide the insertion of a chest drain. Its use requires a fairly significant force.

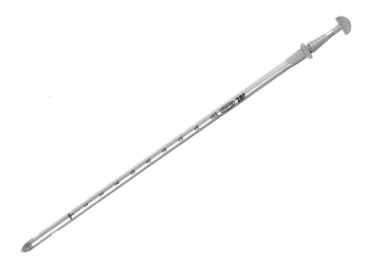

Figure 5.2   Trocar. *Courtesy of Smiths Medical.*

What Are the Indications?

The indications are the same as those for a chest drain insertion. Some clinicians believe that using a trocar will speed up the procedure.

What Are the Contraindications?

Studies have shown that using a trocar rather than a blunt dissection technique with a guidewire causes more injury to anatomical structures and vital organs. Many believe that inserting a chest drain using a trocar is becoming an obsolete technique. The Seldinger technique has by and large superseded the use of a trocar.

What Are the Complications?

Damage to vital organs and nearby structures. Misplacement of the tube. Research has shown that using a trocar is associated with a higher rate of re-expansion pulmonary oedema.

Underwater Seal Device

What Is This?

This is an underwater seal device used for the effective drainage of air or fluid from the pleural space (Figure 5.3). It is a system where the chest tube is placed underwater at a depth with suction applied to a side ventilator port so that air drained from a pneumothorax can be seen as bubbling underwater or fluid drained can be measured in the case of pleural effusions or haemothoraces.

What Are the Indications?

The main indication is for a chest drain as aforementioned. It creates an airtight system to prevent trapping of air or fluids into the pleural cavity. It also allows the monitoring of drainage. The continuous bubbling may mean a visceral pleural air leak or that the tube site has been moved to a point in contact with air.

What Are the Contraindications?

The system should be managed by personnel trained to use the device. It is not suitable as a device to be managed outside the hospital setting.

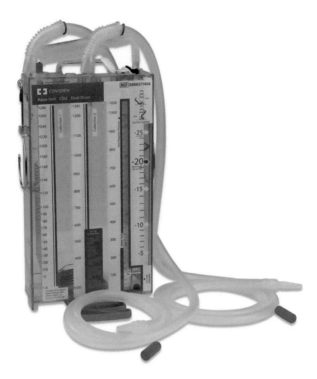

Figure 5.3   Underwater Seal Device. © *2018 courtesy of Cardinal Health UK Ltd.*

What Are the Complications, If Any?

Risk of failure of the device. Risk of positioning error or tipping over of the bottle thereby misplacing the tube ending. If the device is raised above the patient's level, retrograde flow can occur. Patient's mobility is also reduced.

Further Reading

1. Carney M, Ravin CE. Intercostal artery laceration during thoracocentesis: Increased risk in elderly patients. *Chest.* 1979;75(4):520–2. PubMed PMID: 446149.
2. Cha KC, Kim H, Ji HJ, Kwon WC, Shin HJ, Cha YS, Lee KH, Hwang SO, Lee CC, Singer AJ. The frequency of reexpansion pulmonary edema after trocar and hemostat assisted thoracostomy in patients with spontaneous pneumothorax. *Yonsei Med J.* 2013;54(1):166–71. doi: 10.3349/ymj.2013.54.1.166. PubMed PMID: 23225814; PubMed Central PMCID: PMC3521265.
3. Havelock T, Teoh R, Laws D, Gleeson F. BTS Pleural Disease Guideline Group. Pleural procedures and thoracic ultrasound: British Thoracic Society Pleural Disease Guideline 2010. *Thorax.* 2010;65 Suppl 2:ii61–76. doi: 10.1136/thx.2010.137026. PubMed PMID: 20696688.
4. Henry M, Arnold T, Harvey J; Pleural Diseases Group, Standards of Care Committee, British Thoracic Society. BTS guidelines for the management of spontaneous pneumothorax. *Thorax.* 2003;58 Suppl 2:ii39–52. PubMed PMID: 12728149; PubMed Central PMCID: PMC1766020.
5. Laws D, Neville E, Duffy J; Pleural Diseases Group, Standards of Care Committee, British Thoracic Society. BTS guidelines for the insertion of a chest drain. *Thorax.* 2003;58 Suppl 2:ii53–9. PubMed PMID: 12728150; PubMed Central PMCID: PMC1766017.
6. Mahfood S, Hix WR, Aaron BL, Blaes P, Watson DC. Reexpansion pulmonary edema. *Ann Thorac Surg.* 1988;45(3):340–5. Review. PubMed PMID: 3279931.
7. Munnell ER. Thoracic drainage. *Ann Thorac Surg.* 1997;63(5):1497–502. Review. PubMed PMID: 9146363.

EAR, NOSE AND THROAT

6

1) Nasal Speculum
2) Self-Retaining Nasal Speculum
3) Rigid Nasal Endoscope
4) Flexible Nasolaryngoscope

Nasal Speculum

What Is This?

This is a Thudicum nasal speculum (Figure 6.1). It has many sizes to fit adults and children. It is pressed using the index and middle fingers before inserting into the nostril where the prongs are released to visualise the nasal cavity.

What Are the Indications?

They are used for a variety of nasal procedures. These include anterior rhinoscopy, examination and retrieval of superficial foreign bodies, nasal packing and nasal operations such as septoplasty.

What Are the Contraindications?

Patient refusal especially when patient cooperation is important. Conditions such as furunculosis and vestibulitis may render it too painful to proceed.

What Are the Complications, If Any?

These are rare but include pain and minor trauma.

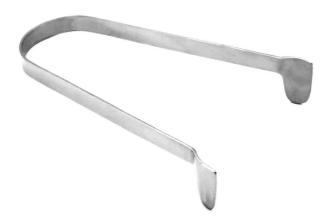

Figure 6.1   Nasal Speculum (Thudicum Nasal Speculum). *Courtesy of Steris Healthcare.*

Nasal Speculum (Self-Retaining)

What Is This?

This is a nasal speculum which has a self-retaining function (Figures 6.2 and 6.3). It comes in different sizes. It is inserted in the nose closed and the two blades are then opened to visualise the nasal cavity. It contains a set screw offering a locking mechanism which frees up the operator's hand.

What Are the Indications?

It can be used for a wide variety of nasal procedures. These include anterior rhinoscopy, nasal packing, septoplasty, polypectomy, examination and retrieval of foreign body and turbinate reduction.

What Are the Contraindications?

Patient refusal especially when patient cooperation is important in nasal examination.

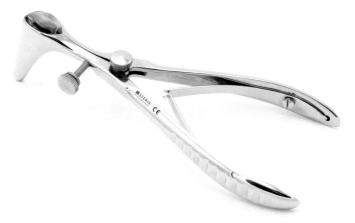

Figure 6.2   Self-Retaining Nasal Speculum (Killian Nasal Speculum). *Courtesy of Steris Healthcare.*

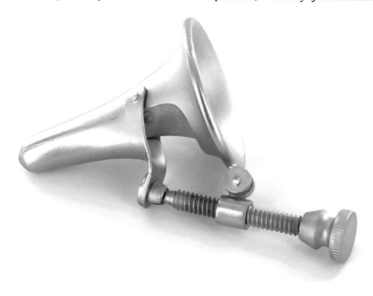

Figure 6.3   Self-Retaining Nasal Speculum (Voltolini Nasal Speculum). *Courtesy of Medema.*

What Are the Complications, If Any?

These are rare but can include pain and minor trauma.

Rigid Nasal Endoscope

What Is This?

This is a rigid nasal endoscope/sinuscope used for nasal rhinoscopy (Figure 6.4). It is a rigid, fibre-optic tube which is connected to a light source where the practitioner can visualise structures directly. It can also be connected to a screen where the practitioner can capture and record images. It is inserted into the nostril to examine the nasal cavity through to the nasopharynx. Before insertion, a topical anaesthetic is used to numb the area and prevent sneezing. Nasal decongestants are usually given to reduce any nasal membrane swelling to ease passage of the endoscope. It is usually done as an outpatient procedure.

What Are the Indications?

These can be divided into diagnostic and therapeutic depending on the model used but it is worth noting that one of the most common indications for nasal endoscopy is investigation for rhinosinusitis.

Other diagnostic indications include any nasal or sinus symptoms that require further examination. These include nasal congestion, facial pressure, long-term discharge/rhinorrhoea, pain and epistaxis. It can also be used for the surveillance of previously diagnosed tumours or polyps within the nasal cavity and paranasal sinuses, biopsy of any abnormal masses as well as investigating a cerebrospinal fluid (CSF) leak, Eustachian tube problems and a loss of smell sensation.

Therapeutically, it can be used for the treatment of epistaxis, retrieval or foreign bodies, irrigation and balloon dilatation of sinuses. It is also used during functional endoscopic sinus surgery (FESS).

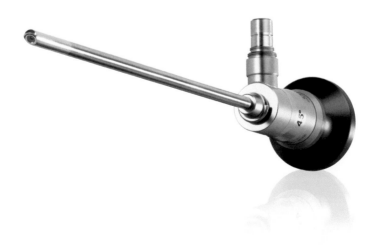

Figure 6.4   Rigid Nasal Endoscope. *Copyright by Olympus Winter & Ibe GmbH.*

What Are the Contraindications?

Patient refusal, especially when patient cooperation is important given the nature of the procedure. Depending on the indication of the procedure, patients may need to stop their anticoagulants prior to it.

What Are the Complications?

These are rare and include pain, bleeding and minor mucosal trauma. More rarely, patients may faint or react to the topical anaesthetic/decongestant.

Flexible Rhinolaryngoscope

What Is This?

This is a flexible fibreoptic/video endoscope used for rhinolaryngoscopy (Figure 6.5). It comes in various sizes from 1.9 mm for children to 6 mm for adults. It has a light source and structures can be visualised directly under the endoscope with a viewing camera attached to the viewing port of the scope or projected on a screen with recording functions. It is usually inserted nasally to visualise the nasopharyngeal anatomy. Depending on the indications, it can be inserted with topical anaesthetic with or without sedation.

What Are the Indications?

In otorhinolaryngology, it is mainly used to perform a flexible nasopharyngoscopy to examine the anatomical structures of the nasal cavity and to visualise any abnormalities such as polyps, foreign bodies and masses. It can also be extended to the nasopharynx and adenoids where any abnormal growth can be examined and biopsied. Further distally, the hypopharynx can be visualised where potential airway obstruction from foreign bodies, obstructive sleep apnoea and abnormal masses can be examined. Dysphonia and dysphagia can also be investigated this way.

What Are the Contraindications?

Acute epiglottitis, when stimulated, can result in laryngospasm which could lead to respiratory compromise and death.

Relative contraindications include:

Coagulopathy: bleeding risk.

Craniofacial trauma: intracranial extension of the endoscope.

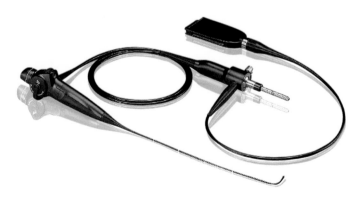

Figure 6.5   Flexible Nasolaryngoscope. *Copyright by Olympus Europa SE & Co. KG.*

What Are the Complications?

There are rare but include bleeding, pain, infection and a hoarse voice post-procedure. There is also a small risk of allergic reaction to the topical anaesthetic or sedative used.

Further Reading

1. Alvi S, Lasrado S. Flexible nasopharyngoscopy. [Updated 2019 Mar 20]. StatPearls [Internet]. Treasure Island, FL: StatPearls Publishing; 2019 Jan. Available from https://www.ncbi.nlm.nih.gov/books/NBK539740/
2. Sargi Z, Casiano R. Endoscopic sinus surgery in patients receiving anticoagulant or antiplatelet therapy. *Am J Rhinol.* 2007;21(3):335–8. PubMed PMID: 17621820.

GENERAL SURGERY

7

1) Hand-Held Abdominal Retractor
2) Self-Retaining Abdominal Retractor
3) Anoscope/Proctoscope
4) Rigid Sigmoidoscope
5) Flexible Sigmoidoscope
6) Colonoscope
7) Tru-Cut Biopsy Device
8) Electrosurgery Electrodes
9) Skin Stapler
10) Needle Holder
11) Sutures
12) Laparoscopic Trocar
13) Laparoscopic Grasper

Hand-Held Abdominal Retractor

What Is This?

This is a hand-held abdominal retractor used to retract the body wall (Figure 7.1). The blade is curved with a blunt end to minimise trauma. It comes in various sizes and may come with a grip handle to be held by a surgical assistant or a flat handle to be attached to a frame and held into position. It is commonly used to hold the abdominal wall open during abdominal or thoracic operations.

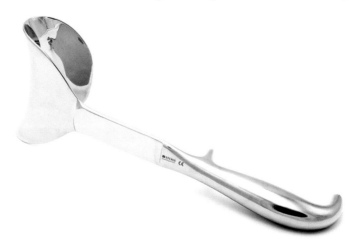

Figure 7.1   Hand-Held Abdominal Retractor. *Courtesy of Steris Healthcare.*

What Are the Indications?

It is most commonly used for laparotomy for various indications including perforated bowels and bowel obstruction. It may also be used in thoracic surgery when the abdominal wall needs to be retracted.

What Are the Contraindications?

There are no absolute contraindications.

What Are the Complications?

These are very rare and appear to occur more often in self-retaining retractors. The most common type of injury is damage to the femoral, iliohypogastric, genito-femoral and ilioinguinal nerves.

Self-Retaining Abdominal Retractor

What Is This?

This is a self-retaining abdominal retractor (Figures 7.2 and 7.3). It comes in various sizes and is used in laparotomy without the need for an assistant to hold the abdomen open with a manual retractor. It has at least two blades which can be locked into place and adjusted to suit the extent of spread needed in order to visualise abdominal contents.

What Are the Indications?

It is indicated in abdominal surgery where examination of abdominal contents or a prolonged operating time is needed. These may include laparotomy for suspected bowel perforation and vascular surgery such as abdominal aortic aneurysm rupture repair.

What Are the Contraindications?

These are relative. Retractors that use a ratchet system are limited by the depth of the blades. In patients of higher BMI, this would mean that another retractor may be needed to retract deeper structures.

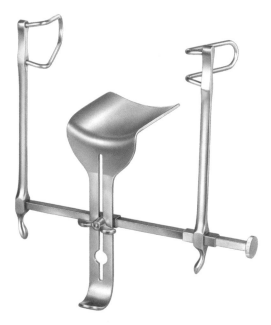

Figure 7.2 Self-Retaining Abdominal Retractor. *Courtesy of KLS Martin.*

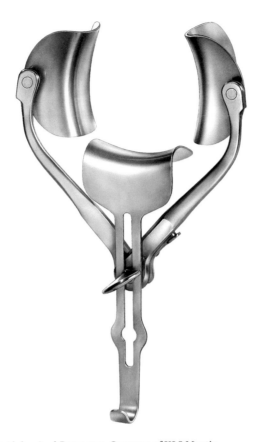

Figure 7.3   Self-Retaining Abdominal Retractor. *Courtesy of KLS Martin.*

There are reports showing that a high BMI, immunosuppression and a history of symptomatic diverticulitis are risk factors for compressive retractor injury.

What Are the Complications?

These are very rare and are generally related to the technique used.

These include vascular, gastrointestinal and neurological complications.

Vascular: Subcapsular haematoma of the liver, small and large bowel ischaemia due to damage to collateral vessels.

Gastrointestinal: Perforation and superficial bowel injury.

Neurological: Iatrogenic nerve injury including femoral and sciatic neuropathies.

Anoscope/Proctoscope

What Is This?

This is an anoscope/proctoscope (Figures 7.4, 7.5 and 7.6). It is a rigid, straight, hollow tube with an inner obturator made from plastic or metal. Some anoscopes/proctoscopes have a light source attached and others will need an external light. It is inserted through the anal passage of the patient to examine the anus (anoscope) and rectum (proctoscope) under direct vision.

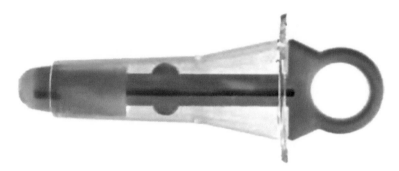

Figure 7.4   Anoscope. *Courtesy of Medema.*

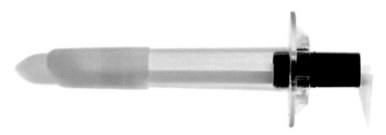

Figure 7.5   Proctoscope/Rectoscope. *Courtesy of Medema.*

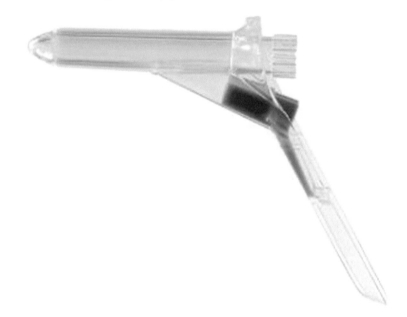

Figure 7.6   Proctoscope/Rectoscope. *Courtesy of Medema.*

What Are the Indications?

These are divided into investigative and therapeutic.

Investigative: It is indicated when examination of the anal passage and rectum is needed. These can include evaluation of rectal bleeding for suspected haemorrhoids or perianal pathology, anal pain/discharge/prolapse, perianal ulcers/itching, masses felt on digital rectal examination and suspected foreign bodies. It can also be used to obtain biopsies of suspected lesions and samples for microbiology to investigate suspected sexually transmitted infections (STIs).

Therapeutic: These may include retrieval of foreign body and treatment of internal haemorrhoids by rubber band ligation.

What Are the Contraindications?

Patient refusal and imperforate/resected anus would contraindicate the procedure. Immunosuppressed patients should not have a digital rectal examination/anoscopy done due to the risk of infection. Depending on the proposed procedure, coagulopathy may contraindicate the procedure.

What Are the Complications?

These are rare and depend on what procedures have been performed. They can be classified as immediate, early and late complications.

Immediate: Patients may experience some discomfort and feel the need for defecation. Bleeding may occur if the mucosa has been damaged.

Early: Infection, urinary retention, bleeding and severe pain may occur especially when a rubber band ligation has been done.

Late: Recurrence of haemorrhoids/failure of the therapeutic procedure and failure to diagnose cancerous/precancerous lesions.

Rigid Sigmoidoscope

What Is This?

This is a rigid sigmoidoscope (Figure 7.7). It is a 25 cm, straight, hollow scope made from metal or plastic with an air insufflation handle and a light source attached allowing direct visualisation of parts of the colon. There are single-use and reusable versions. A digital rectal examination should always be performed beforehand. It is then inserted into the rectum and sigmoid colon through the anus of a patient primarily for examination purposes with or without therapeutic intervention. It is less commonly done than flexible sigmoidoscopy and is usually done as an outpatient procedure often on unprepared bowels.

What Are the Indications?

These can be divided into investigative and therapeutic.

Investigative: It is indicated when examination of the colon up to the sigmoid is needed. This may be for bowel screening in some cases. Other indications could be investigation for suspected anorectal ulcers and cancer, rectal bleeding, non-specific proctitis and iron-deficiency/unexplained anaemia. Biopsies can also be taken during the procedure.

Therapeutic: Usually done alongside an investigative sigmoidoscopy and include polypectomy, achieving haemostasis in the case of bleeding and conservative management of sigmoid volvulus.

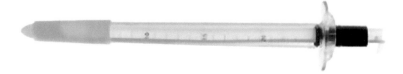

Figure 7.7   Rigid Sigmoidoscope. *Courtesy of Medema.*

What Are the Contraindications?

Patients with confirmed or suspected bowel perforation should not have a rigid sigmoidoscopy. Other contraindications include bowel infarction, acute peritonitis, toxic megacolon and acute severe diverticulitis. Patients with current cardiac arrhythmia and myocardial ischaemia should have cardiac monitoring during the procedure. Postponement of the procedure until the conditions are optimised should be considered. It is generally contraindicated in patients with coagulopathy and neutropaenia given the risk of bleeding and infection, respectively.

What Are the Complications?

These are divided into immediate, early and late.

Immediate: Bowel perforation, bleeding, pain and discomfort.

Early: Bleeding, infection, diarrhoea, vomiting, pain, discomfort and polypectomy coagulation syndrome.

Late: Missed diagnosis of malignant or precancerous lesions.

Flexible Sigmoidoscope

What Is This?

This is a flexible sigmoidoscope (Figure 7.8). It is a flexible fibre-optic endoscope of a typical length of 60 cm with an air insufflation handle and a light source attached to allow visualisation of parts of the colon. It is inserted into the patient, usually in the left lateral position, through the anus primarily for examination purposes with or without therapeutic intervention. It offers a greater range of viewing angles owing to the flexibility and the possibility of tip deflection. It has advantages over rigid sigmoidoscopy because of the possibility of a more extensive examination of the distal colon and hence a higher sensitivity in picking up colorectal cancer and precancerous lesions. It is also better tolerated by patients given its higher comfort levels. The disadvantage of a flexible sigmoidoscopy is the need for bowel preparation.

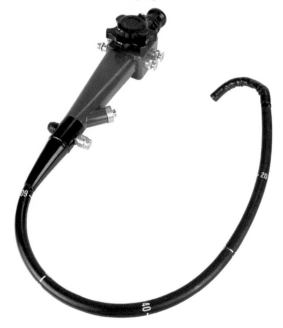

Figure 7.8 Flexible Sigmoidoscope. *Courtesy of A1MedTech.*

What Are the Indications?

These can be divided into investigative and therapeutic.

Investigative: It is indicated when examination of the colon up to the sigmoid is needed. This could be for bowel screening programmes for patients above the age of 50–55 that is being introduced in the UK and for patients with a family history of familial adenomatous polyposis (FAP). Other purposes could be investigation for unintentional weight loss, rectal bleeding, iron-deficiency/unexplained anaemia and surveillance post-resection of rectal tumours. Biopsies can also be taken during the procedure.

Therapeutic: These include polypectomy, foreign body retrieval, dilatation of benign rectal stenosis, endoscopic mucosal resection and achieving haemostasis in the case of bleeding.

What Are the Contraindications?

Patients with an acute abdomen including known or suspected bowel perforation, acute diverticulitis and fulminant colitis should not have the procedure done. Other contraindications include patient refusal, uncooperative patient and inadequate bowel preparation. Patients with current cardiac arrhythmia and myocardial ischaemia should have cardiac monitoring during the procedure. Postponement of the procedure until the conditions are optimised should be considered.

What Are the Complications?

These are divided into immediate, early and late.

Immediate: Bowel perforation, bleeding, pain and discomfort.

Early: Bleeding, infection, pain, discomfort and polypectomy coagulation syndrome.

Late: Missed diagnosis of malignant or precancerous lesions.

Colonoscope

What Is This?

This is a colonoscope (Figure 7.9). It is a fibre-optic, flexible, thin tube that is used for the examination of the entire colon. It has a light source, a light bundle, a proximal handle, an instrument channel, a water/air channel and, depending on the model, a camera at the distal end or a fibre-optic camera

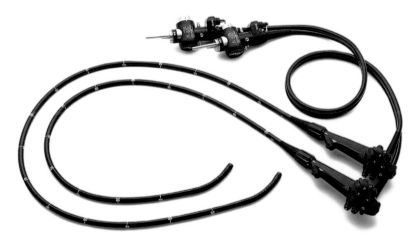

Figure 7.9   Colonoscope. *Copyright by Olympus Europa SE & Co. KG.*

at the proximal end to visualise the colon. It is inserted into a patient's colon, typically in the left lateral position, through the anal passage. It is capable of examining the entire large colon up to the caecum. Bowel preparation is needed before a colonoscopy.

The advantages of colonoscopy over sigmoidoscopy is the more extensive examination of the entire large bowel thereby making it more sensitive in picking up abnormalities.

What Are the Indications?

These can be divided into investigative and therapeutic.

Investigative: It is indicated when examination of the entire colon is needed. The most common indications are the screening and investigation for colorectal cancer. These include bowel screening for patients above the age of 50 in many countries and for patients with a family history of Lynch syndrome. Other purposes could be investigation for unintentional weight loss, rectal bleeding, iron deficiency/unexplained anaemia and surveillance post-resection of tumours/polyps. Biopsies can also be taken during the procedure.

Therapeutic: These include polypectomy, endoscopic mucosal resection, endoscopic colonic decompression +/– stenting, dilatation of benign colonic stenosis, retrieval of foreign bodies and achieving haemostasis in the case of bleeding.

What Are the Contraindications?

It is generally contraindicated in patients with an acute abdomen including known or suspected bowel perforation, acute diverticulitis and fulminant colitis. Other contraindications include patient refusal, uncooperative patient and inadequate bowel preparation. Patients with current cardiac arrhythmia and myocardial ischaemia should have cardiac monitoring during the procedure. Postponement of the procedure until the conditions are optimised should be considered.

What Are the Complications?

These are divided into immediate, early and late.

Immediate: Bowel perforation, bleeding, pain and discomfort.

Early: Bleeding, infection, pain, discomfort and polypectomy coagulation syndrome.

Late: Missed diagnosis of malignant or precancerous lesions.

Tru-Cut Biopsy Device

What Is This?

This is a Tru-Cut biopsy device (Figure 7.10). It is used to obtain tissue samples from a patient with minimal trauma. It consists of a scalpel-sharp cutting edge at the tip, a more proximal 20 mm specimen notch to retrieve the sample and a removable stylet to enable multiple sampling.

What Are the Indications?

It is used for the biopsy of body tissues for investigative purposes. The applicable settings range from percutaneous biopsy of the liver and breast to endoscopic ultrasound-guided Tru-Cut biopsy of the gastrointestinal tract and CT-guided lytic bone biopsy.

What Are the Contraindications?

There are general and site-dependent contraindications.

General: Coagulopathy, thrombocytopaenia, patient refusal and uncooperative patient.

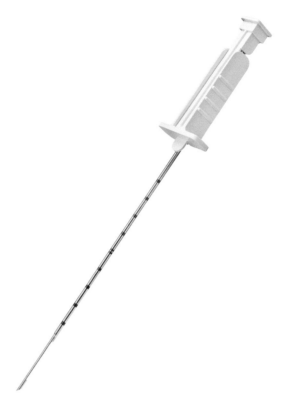

Figure 7.10   Tru-Cut Biopsy Device. *Courtesy of Merit Medical UK.*

Site-specific examples: In some cases, percutaneous liver biopsy may be contraindicated in tense non-resolving ascites and patients with a high BMI when prior paracentesis or the transjugular method is preferred. Other contraindications include haemangioma, extrahepatic biliary obstruction and bacterial cholangitis.

What Are the Complications?

These are divided into immediate, early and late which are also divided into general and site-specific.

Immediate:

General: Pain, bleeding, damage to the nearby/underlying structures, hypotension and vasovagal episodes.

Specific: For example, significant haemorrhage from punctured haematomas can occur in percutaneous liver biopsy. Other complications include puncturing the lung, gallbladder and colon, haemobilia, subcutaneous emphysema and pneumothorax.

Early:

General: Infection, pain, ecchymosis and sepsis.

Specific: For example, biliary peritonitis followed by biliary puncture in liver biopsy and haemobilia.

Late:

General: Scarring.

Specific: Intrahepatic arteriovenous fistulae in percutaneous liver biopsy.

Electrosurgery Electrodes

What Is This?

This is an electrosurgery electrode (Figures 7.11 through 7.13). Electrosurgery refers to the conversion of electric current to high frequency alternating current (HFAC) using a diathermy machine, which is then used on body tissues. There are 3 main effects of electrosurgery on the body: cutting, desiccation and fulguration. The setting used depends on whether the desired effect is to coagulate, vaporise or dehydrate tissues as a means of destruction.

There are two types of electrosurgery: monopolar and bipolar. The monopolar blade delivers the HFAC through an electrode into the patient's body which then returns to the diathermy machine through a pad attached to another part of the patient's body. The bipolar blade, on the other hand, has two blades which are used to grasp the patient's tissue to form a complete circuit of the HFAC. The monopolar technique is more versatile but also poses a higher risk of burns. The bipolar technique allows the electrical energy to be focussed on a particular part of the tissue without the need for a return pad, thereby reducing the risk and maximising efficiency. The monopolar form

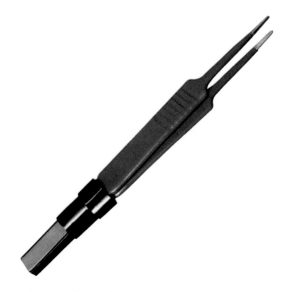

Figure 7.11   Electrosurgery Electrodes (Bipolar). *Courtesy of Accrington Surgical Ltd.*

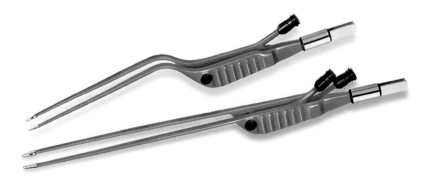

Figure 7.12   Electrosurgery Electrodes (Bipolar). *Courtesy of KLS Martin.*

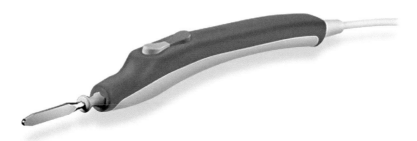

Figure 7.13   Electrosurgery Electrodes (Monopolar). *Courtesy of KLS Martin.*

uses a single blade. The bipolar technique uses a double blade. The advantage of electrosurgery is that it makes surgery more efficient thereby reducing anaesthetic time.

What Are the Indications?

There are many indications. Electrosurgery may be used in procedures that require cutting and coagulation. These can range from eye, dental, dermatological to general surgical, endoscopic and laparoscopic procedures.

What Are the Contraindications?

Electrosurgery may interfere with implanted cardiac devices including pacemakers and implantable cardiac defibrillators (ICDs). Depending on the device, settings and indications, pacemakers may have to be temporarily switched to an asynchronous pacing mode and the ICD temporarily inactivated due to potential "electrical noise" from the electrosurgical currents. Laparoscopic electrosurgery creates a risk for an alternate path to earth; the equipment used should have insulation properties.

What Are the Complications?

These are wide-ranging and may be specific to the sites and techniques used. They can be divided into immediate, early and late. It should, however, be noted that burns and fires are major risks of electrosurgery. Alternate site burns may also happen if an alternate path to earth through other sites of the body is established. The risk of deep tissue burns is proportional to the time under electrosurgery and the current used. The greater the area of the return electrode, the lesser the risk.

Immediate: Burns, alternate site burns, shocks, infection transmission and pacemaker/ICD malfunction.

Early: In the case of dermatological surgery, there is a risk of delayed bleeding as well as infectious and non-infectious complications from smoke plume inhalation.

Late: In the case of dermatological surgery, there is a risk of scarring with hyperpigmentation.

Skin Stapler

What Is This?

This is a skin stapler (Figure 7.14). It is a single-use instrument for wound closure. It dispenses one staple each time the trigger is activated. The staple penetrates the skin and holds the wound closed.

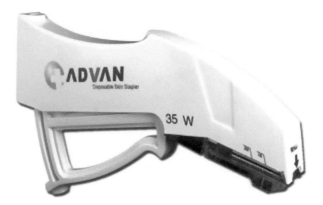

Figure 7.14 Skin Stapler. *Courtesy of Medema.*

What Are the Indications?

It is used for the closure of wounds and incisions of the skin. This may encompass a wide variety of procedures including laparotomy.

What Are the Contraindications?

Hypersensitivity to the material. It should not be used on the face, head and neck given the cosmetic consequences. It should not be used on the hands and feet given the discomfort and inconvenience posed on day-to-day activities of the patient. It should be avoided in patients who may need MRI as the staples may be avulsed in the magnetic field.

What Are the Complications?

These are classified as immediate, early and late.

Immediate: Failure to form a closed staple, puncturing the underlying structures if a certain distance is not maintained between the skin and the delicate structures underneath.

Early: Embedded staples and wound dehiscence.

Late: Hypertrophic scarring.

Needle Holder

What Is this?

This is a needle holder (Figures 7.15 and 7.16). The diamond jaw ensures a secure grasp of surgical needles.

What Are the Indications?

Holding a suturing needle for wound closure.

What Are the Contraindications?

None.

What Are the Complications?

Suture snagging. Microtrauma on tissues if misused.

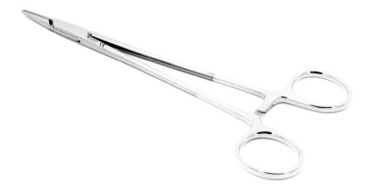

Figure 7.15   Needle Holder. *Courtesy of Steris Healthcare.*

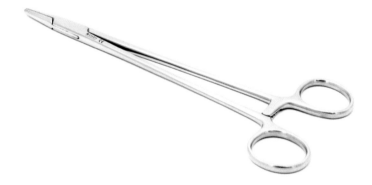

Figure 7.16   Needle Holder. *Courtesy of Steris Healthcare.*

Sutures

What Is This?

This is a surgical suture (Figures 7.17 through 7.19). It is used to repair body issues through healing facilitation. It usually comes as a single unit with a needle attached to the end of the suture. It is held at the needle about one third of the way above the suture using a needle holder. The type of needle used depends on the target tissue. A tapered needle should not be used on the skin due to the difficulty in skin penetration; a cutting needle should be used instead.

Sutures can be broadly divided into absorbable or non-absorbable materials. Either material can be natural or synthetic in nature.

Absorbable natural	Catgut
Absorbable synthetic	Vicryl, Monocryl
Non-absorbable natural	Cotton, Silk
Non-absorbable synthetic	Prolene, Nylon

Natural absorbable sutures are made from animal intestines and are broken down by enzymatic reaction within 1–3 weeks depending on whether they have been collagen treated. Synthetic absorbable

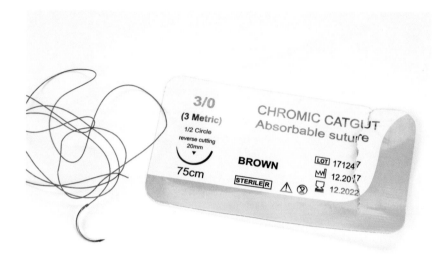

Figure 7.17   Sutures.

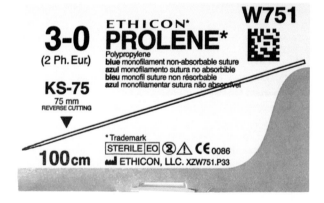

Figure 7.18   Sutures.

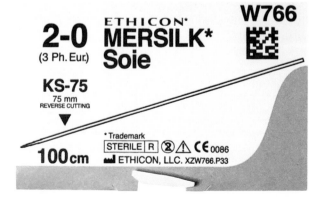

Figure 7.19   Sutures.

sutures are made from polymers which are broken down by hydrolysis in 3–8 weeks depending on the material used. Non-absorbable sutures, on the other hand, do not break down naturally. They are either left in place indefinitely or taken out when adequate healing has taken place.

Sutures can be further subdivided into monofilament and multifilament. Monofilament sutures, as its name suggests, are single-stranded whereas multifilament sutures are made from multi-stranded fibres which makes it easier to handle due to increased friction. This increased friction, however, also increases the damage to body tissues during the suturing process.

Non-absorbable sutures in the skin require removal on healing. The following site-specific timetable is a guide to when sutures should be removed.

Suture removal:

Face 3–4 days

Scalp 5 days

Trunk 7 days

Arm and leg 7–10 days

Foot 10–14 days

What Are the Indications?

These are wide-ranging and can include many parts of the body. These may include simple skin lacerations, vascular repair, intestinal anastomosis, skin grafts and flaps, closure of surgical incisions and nerve repair.

What Are the Contraindications?

Hypersensitivity to the specific suture materials. A highly contaminated wound may be best left open rather than closed by sutures. The type of suture should be carefully chosen taking into account the site and indication of use.

What Are the Complications?

These are divided into immediate, early and late. They can also be related to complications of suture removal.

Immediate: Snagging of the suture, bending of the needle if held too close to the base, excess trauma to the body tissue and damage to the nearby structures including the viscera and delicate organs.

Early: Suture reaction including inflammation, unhealed wound, wound reopening/breakdown and infection.

Late: Suture spitting, suture tracking, stitch abscess, granulation, fistula, fibrosis and hypertrophic scarring.

Laparoscopic Port

What Is This?

This is a laparoscopic port (Figure 7.20). It is a pen-shaped laparoscopic instrument with a sharp end which is encased by a sleeve/cannula. It is inserted through the skin to create a surgical opening into the body cavity. The trocar is then removed leaving the cannula/sleeve in situ providing surgical

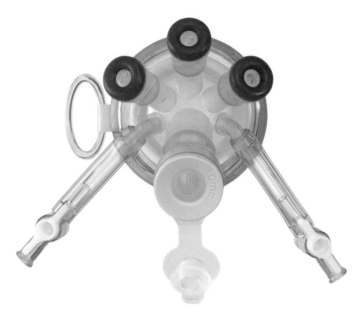

Figure 7.20   Laparoscopic Port. *Copyright by Olympus Winter & Ibe GmbH.*

access to the site of operation laparoscopically whilst sealing the skin. It makes laparoscopic surgery possible by providing access to surgical equipment including laparoscopes, graspers and electrosurgical electrodes. It also allows the removal of body tissues including biopsy samples.

What Are the Indications?

These are wide-ranging but can be divided into investigative and therapeutic.

Investigative: Exploratory laparoscopy may be indicated in non-specific abdominal pain where typical diagnostic and radiological means have not yielded a diagnosis. It may also be indicated in haemodynamically stable trauma patients who are suspected to have sustained abdominal injuries. In certain upper-gastrointestinal cancers such as that of the oesophagus, staging laparoscopy is indicated if radical surgery is being planned. Other indications for a diagnostic laparoscopy include chronic pelvic pain and liver disease otherwise non-specific on radiological scans.

Therapeutic: These include tumour resection and appendicectomy.

What Are the Contraindications?

Absolute contraindications to a diagnostic laparoscopy include pathologies that require therapeutic interventions such as bowel perforation, acute obstruction and known intra-abdominal trauma.

Other contraindications to laparoscopy in general include uncorrected coagulopathy/thrombocytopaenia, extensive intra-abdominal adhesions, suspected abdominal compartment syndrome and a recent laparotomy.

What Are the Complications?

There are a number of factors that may cause complications in a laparoscopy. These include consequences from the laparoscopic instruments, the physiological changes from pneumoperitoneum and positioning.

Laparoscopic Instruments: Vascular and visceral injury, bleeding and scarring.

Pneumoperitoneum: Venous gas embolism, vagal stimulation > bradycardia + asystole, raised intraabdominal pressure > compression of the inferior vena cava > reduced preload > decreased cardiac output, splinting of the diaphragm > reduced lung compliance > hypoxaemia, increased CO_2 intraabdominally > hypercarbia > increased intracranial pressure (ICP).

Positioning: Trendelenburg position > raised ICP + further splinting of the diaphragm and hypoxaemia/hypercarbia. Reverse Trendelenburg > reduced preload > hypotension. Very rarely, the Trendelenburg position may cause "Well Leg Compartment Syndrome" due to reduced perfusion and venous drainage.

Laparoscopic Grasper

What Is This?

This is a laparoscopic grasper (Figures 7.21 and 7.22). It has a rotatable and flexible/rigid shaft, and double-action blunt jaws. It can come with bipolar or insulation capabilities.

What Are the Indications?

They are used in laparoscopic procedures. Depending on the exactly model, it can be used in electrosurgery as electrodes and monopolar cautery as well as mobilising tissues and obtaining a specimen or biopsy samples.

What Are the Contraindications?

There is no absolute contraindication to using laparoscopic graspers. If used as electrosurgery, the currents may interfere with implanted cardiac devices including pacemakers and implantable cardiac defibrillators (ICD). Depending on the actual model, settings and indications, pacemakers may have to be temporarily switched to an asynchronous pacing mode and ICD temporarily inactivated due to potential "electrical noise" from the electrosurgical currents.

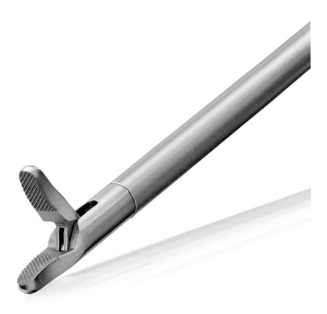

Figure 7.21 Laparoscopic Grasper. *Copyright by Olympus Europa SE & Co. KG.*

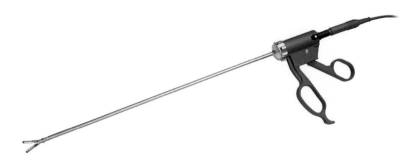

Figure 7.22   Laparoscopic Grasper. *Courtesy of KLS Martin.*

What Are the Complications?

These include dropping the specimen and tearing the grasped tissues.

When used as part of electrosurgery, care should be taken to ensure that instruments with insulation are used to avoid an alternative path of earthing. Thermal injury may cause bowel perforation.

Further Reading

1. Baigrie D, Badri T. Electrosurgery. [Updated 2018 Oct 27]. StatPearls [Internet]. Treasure Island, FL: StatPearls Publishing; 2019 Jan. Available from https://www.ncbi.nlm.nih.gov/books/NBK48 2380/

2. Benoit G, Moukarzel M, Verdelli G, Hiesse C, Buffet C, Bensadoun H, Charpentier B, Jardin A, Fries D. Gastrointestinal complications in renal transplantation. *Transpl Int.* 1993;6(1):45–9. PubMed PMID: 8452632.

3. Kim JW, Shin SS. Ultrasound-guided percutaneous core needle biopsy of abdominal viscera: Tips to ensure safe and effective biopsy. *Korean J Radiol.* 2017;18(2):309–322. doi: 10.3348/kjr.2017.18.2.309. Epub 2017 Feb 7. PubMed PMID: 28246511; PubMed Central PMCID: PMC5313519.

4. Kukreja A. *Anorectal Surgery Made Easy.* JP Medical Ltd., 2013; ISBN 935025719X, 9789350257197.

5. Noldus J, Graefen M, Huland H. Major postoperative complications secondary to use of the Bookwalter self-retaining retractor. *Urology.* 2002;60(6):964–7. PubMed PMID: 12475650.

6. Perugini RA, Callery MP. Complications of laparoscopic surgery. In: Holzheimer RG, Mannick JA, editors. *Surgical Treatment: Evidence-Based and Problem-Oriented.* Munich: Zuckschwerdt; 2001. Available from https://www.ncbi.nlm.nih.gov/books/NBK6923/

7. Pirenne J, Lledo-Garcia E, Benedetti E, West M, Hakim NS, Sutherland DE, Gruessner RW, Najarian JS, Matas AJ. Colon perforation after renal transplantation: A single-institution review. *Clin Transplant.* 1997;11(2):88–93. PubMed PMID: 9113442.

ORTHOPAEDICS

8

1) Cervical Collar
2) Knee Prosthesis
3) Hip Prosthesis
4) Dynamic Hip Screw
5) Neutralisation Plate
6) Buttress Plate
7) Compression Plate
8) Intramedullary Nail
9) Kirchner Wire
10) Orthopaedic Cast

Cervical Collar

What Is This?

This is a cervical collar which keeps the cervical spine in its neutral alignment by restricting any form of neck movement including flexion, extension and rotation (Figure 8.1). It does not,

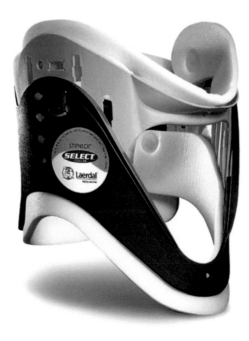

Figure 8.1 Cervical Collar. *Courtesy of Laerdal Medical.*

however, reduce axial loading. Cervical collars can come in various forms and shapes for different purposes. The illustrated cervical collar is often used alongside lateral head blocks and tapes to prevent cervical spine movement in trauma.

What Are the Indications?

These are divided into acute, subacute and chronic.

Acute: Trauma with suspected spinal injury. This should follow the Advanced Trauma Life Support (ATLS) guidelines and be used alongside other immobilisation equipment such as lateral head blocks, tapes and a spine board.

Subacute: Whiplash injuries, acute/repetitive neck injuries and strained neck injuries.

Chronic: Arthritis, cervical radiculopathy and recovery from cervical surgery/fractures.

What Are the Contraindications?

It is contraindicated in patients with a tracheostomy. It should not be used in patients with penetrating neck trauma.

What Are the Complications?

These are divided into early and late.

Early: Discomfort, anxiety, increased intracranial pressure, pain and difficulty to ventilate.

Late: Pressure ulcers/sores, aspiration risk, difficulty weaning off the ventilator if ventilated, general immobility leading to Deep Vein Thrombosis (DVT) and mandibular nerve palsy.

Knee Prosthesis

What Is This?

This is a knee prosthetic implant which is used for a total knee arthroplasty (TKA) (Figure 8.2). It can be made of metal alloys plus ceramic or plastic parts. It has 3 components: the femoral part, the patella part and the tibial component with a plastic spacer. The rationale is to recreate the surfaces of the hinge joint of the knee by first removing damaged bones and/or cartilages and replacing them with metal prostheses and a plastic spacer to ensure better movement and reduce wear and tear. The femoral component has various forms including the posterior-stabilised design, the cruciate-retaining design and the bicruciate-retaining design. The posterior-stabilised design involves removing the cruciate ligaments and replacing it with a centre post-cam design in the prosthesis that substitutes the function of the posterior cruciate ligament. The Cruciate-retaining design requires the retention of the posterior cruciate ligament as it does not offer a substitution. The Bicruciate-retaining design, on the other hand, is a relatively new design that requires the retention of both the anterior and posterior cruciate ligaments with the aim to mimic the human knee as closely as possible.

The tibial component also has 2 main designs: fixed-bearing and mobile-bearing. The fixed bearing design, as its name suggests, has the polyethylene part firmly fixed onto the metal part beneath it. The mobile-bearing part, on the other hand, allows the polyethylene component to

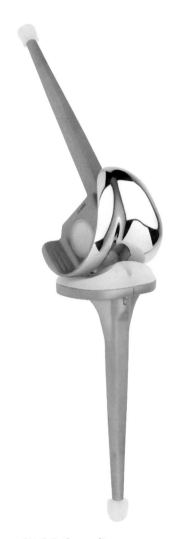

Figure 8.2   Knee Prosthesis. *Courtesy of Link Orthopaedics.*

rotate short distances within the metal tibial tray. This serves as an advantage over the fixed-bearing design by reducing wear and tear. Most TKA prostheses last around 25 years.

What Are the Indications?

The primary indication for TKA is arthritis-related knee pain leading to impaired day-to-day function and/or sleep disturbance. The most common cause is osteoarthritis. Other causes include rheumatoid arthritis, osteonecrosis and other inflammatory arthritis. TKA is usually only indicated after conservative and medical measures have been exhausted. Patients should also have radiographic evidence of degenerative joint disease such as narrowed joint space, osteophytes and sclerosis, though the severity of which may not mirror their symptoms and surgery should not be precluded on this basis.

What Are the Contraindications?

Active infection is an absolute contraindication. Severe peripheral arterial disease and absent extensor mechanisms are also contraindications. Other contraindications are relative and include young age, incompliance, overlying skin conditions such as psoriasis and a high BMI. Co-morbidities may be a significant factor contraindicating the anaesthetic technique proposed which can be regional or general.

What Are the Complications?

These are divided into immediate, early and late.

Immediate: Bleeding, damage to the nearby structures such as nerves and ligaments, periarticular fracture and anaesthetic complications.

Early : Swelling, poor wound healing, wound infection, DVT, haemarthrosis, periprosthetic fracture, prosthetic joint infection and paraesthesia around the scar.

Late: Stiffness of the knee, restricted range of movement, persistent pain, prosthetic joint infection, periprosthetic fracture, excessive scarring and severe heterotopic ossification.

Hip Prosthesis

What Is This?

This is a hip prosthesis used as an implant for hip arthroplasty (Figure 8.3). A total hip prosthesis consists of 3 components: an acetabular component, a femoral component with a head and stem and a plastic liner.

A hip hemiarthroplasty is done through open surgery where the diseased femoral head is removed and replaced with the implant with the femoral stem inserted into the centre of the femur.

In a total hip arthroplasty, the acetabulum is also removed and is replaced with the acetabular component of the prosthesis. This completes the ball and socket prosthetic joint.

What Are the Indications?

The primary indication for a hip replacement is arthritis-related pain. Functional limitation of arthritis is another indication, usually associated with pain. The main cause is osteoarthritis. Other causes include rheumatoid arthritis and any inflammatory joint conditions. Stiffness from conditions such as ankylosing spondylitis is so debilitating that it would warrant a hip replacement even when not associated with pain. Another common indication is hip fracture.

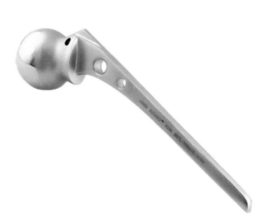

Figure 8.3   Hip Prosthesis. *Courtesy of Biomed Healthtech Ltd.*

What Are the Contraindications?

Absolute contraindications include active joint or systemic infection and invasive tumours that preclude the possibility of adequate fixation of the prosthesis.

Relative contraindications include obesity and young age.

What Are the Complications?

There are divided into immediate, early and late.

Immediate: Bleeding, fracture, discrepancy in leg length, damage to nearby structures such as vessels and nerves, and abductor muscle disruption.

Early: Deep vein thrombosis (DVT), wound infection, delayed wound healing, prosthetic dislocation, paraesthesia, periprosthetic fracture, implant fracture and prosthetic joint infection.

Late: Loosening, dislocation, prosthetic joint infection, heterotopic ossification, implant fracture as well as wear and tear of the prosthesis.

Dynamic Hip Screw

What Is This?

This is a dynamic hip screw (DHS) (Figure 8.4). It consists of a large cancellous lag screw, a metal sleeve attached to a plate and associated screws that fix the plate to the cortex of the femur. The lag screw slides freely into the metal sleeve thereby offering dynamic compression of the

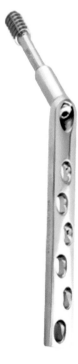

Figure 8.4   Dynamic Hip Screw. *Courtesy of Biomed Healthtech Ltd.*

fracture through transferring weight-bearing forces to the femoral metaphysis. Bone healing and remodelling occur with the maintained reduction of the fracture.

What Are the Indications?

It is used for the internal fixation of proximal femoral fractures. It is mainly indicated in extracapsular fractures such as stable and compressible intertrochanteric hip fractures. It may also be used for intracapsular hip fractures where avascular necrosis is less likely such as those of Garden classification types I and II. Given the high functional demands of younger patients, DHS may still be used for higher-grade fractures in this population to preserve bone stock and avoid complications of replacement arthroplasty such as revision arthroplasty.

What Are the Contraindications?

The dynamic hip screw is intended for compressible and reducible fractures. Fractures that are irreducible or incompressible are therefore contraindicated. Fractures with a high risk of avascular necrosis of the femoral head should contraindicate the use of dynamic hip screws. In these cases, a hip replacement is likely more beneficial.

Other more general contraindications include contraindications to anaesthetics, severe arthritis as well as active systemic and local infections.

What Are the Complications?

These can be divided into immediate, early and late.

Immediate: damage to the nearly structures such as blood vessels and nerves, anaesthetic complications, failure of implant, insufficient reduction and bleeding.

Early: Infection, thromboembolic events, atelectasis, pain, avascular necrosis of the femoral head and screw fracture.

Late: loss of/reduced mobility, residual pain and pseudarthrosis.

Neutralisation Plate

What Is This?

This is a neutralisation plate used for the internal fixation of bone fractures (Figure 8.5). It comes in various sizes and shapes. It acts to protect fracture surfaces from bending, rotating and axial loading. it was developed to protect the fracture site from compression and torsional forces whilst other adjunctives such as lag screws serve to compress the fracture site. It does not itself offer compression to the fracture site. However, newer dynamic compression plates can have various modes including compression and neutralisation (protection). Theoretically, any plate can act as a neutralisation plate if applied to a fracture site in a neutral fashion to withstand bending, compression and torsional forces to the fractured bone.

What Are the Indications?

General indications: To restore anatomical alignment and to provide additional resistance to external forces when screws alone are inadequate.

Specific indications: Any fractures that require neutralisation of bending, compression and rotational forces. These include fibular fractures in the ankle and where inter-fragmentary compression is provided by lag screws but a neutralisation plate is needed to withstand the rotational and bending forces which otherwise would have been inadequate with the lag screws

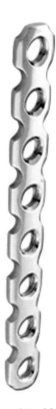

Figure 8.5   Neutralisation Plate. *Courtesy of Biomed Healthtech Ltd.*

alone. Other common indications are wedge fractures of the humerus, radius and ulnar where the neutralisation plate decreases the loading force onto the inter-fragmentary screws.

What Are the Contraindications?

Absolute contraindications include active systemic and local infection, as well as any hypersensitivity to the materials used for the implant. Relative contraindications include severe osteoporosis where adequate fixation may not be possible, patient incompliance and excessive stress on the bone and implant, which may increase the failure rates of the implant.

What Are the Complications?

Immediate:

General: Anaesthetic risks and bleeding.

Specific: Damage to the nearby structures such as nerves, tendons and vessels, failure of the procedure due to insufficient fixation/screw fracture, poor reduction quality and hypersensitivity to the implant materials.

Early:

General: DVT and wound complications such as delayed healing and infection.

Specific: Graft extrusion, plate dislodgement/breakage and neurological symptoms such as paraesthesia.

Late:

General: Scarring.

Specific: Implant-associated infection, distal screw fractures, ossification, malunion, delayed union, stress fracture, pseudarthrosis, cortical necrosis and porosis.

Compression Plate

What Is This?

This is a dynamic compression internal fixation plate (Figure 8.6). It is used to join two bony fragments together with axial compression. It has built-in screw holes that are geometrically designed to offer axial compression when combined with screws. When screws are tightened, the screw heads will glide across the holes thereby moving the plate towards the direction of the fracture resulting in compression. This serves to provide absolute stability to the fracture site to aid bone healing.

What Are the Indications?

It is indicated when bony buttressing at the fracture site is adequate. This includes most simple fractures such as long bone oblique and transverse fractures.

What Are the Contraindications?

Absolute contraindications include active systemic and local infection, as well as any hypersensitivity to the materials used for the implant. Relative contraindications include severe osteoporosis where adequate fixation may not be possible, patient incompliance and excessive stress on the bone and implant, which may increase the failure rates of the implant.

It is contraindicated when bony buttressing is inadequate at the fracture site – these include comminuted fractures and bone loss.

What Are the Complications?

These are divided into immediate, early, late and are subdivided into general and specific.

Immediate:

General: Anaesthetic risks and bleeding.

Specific: Damage to the nearby structures such as nerves, tendons and vessels, failure of the procedure due to insufficient fixation/screw fracture, poor reduction quality and hypersensitivity to the implant materials.

Early:

General: Deep Vein Thrombosis (DVT) and wound complications such as delayed healing and infection.

Specific: Graft extrusion, plate dislodgement/breakage and neurological symptoms such as paraesthesia.

Late:

General: Scarring.

Specific: Implant-associated infection, distal screw fractures, ossification, malunion, delayed union, stress fracture, pseudarthrosis, cortical necrosis and porosis.

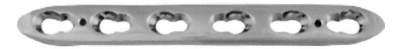

Figure 8.6   Compression Plate. *Courtesy of Innovation Ortho Line Ltd.*

Buttress Plate

What Is This?

This is a buttress plate which is used for the internal fixation of bone fractures (Figure 8.7). It comes in different sizes and special shapes depending on the buttressing requirements. It is thinner than a compression plate. It is carefully contoured to suit the type of fracture in question. It is mainly used to provide support to unstable fractures against compression forces and vertical shear forces during axial loading, especially helpful at articular surfaces such as the ankle and the knee. They are useful for metaphyseal fractures in supporting intra-articular fractures, by preventing the sliding and impaction from the desired position. They are therefore sometimes referred to as periarticular plates.

What Are the Indications?

Fractures at the end of long bones where compressive and axial forces are high. Fractures at articular surfaces, particularly for impacted fractures where elevation to a desired position is needed.

What Are the Contraindications?

These are general. Absolute contraindications include active systemic/local infection and any hypersensitivity to the materials used for the implant. Relative contraindications include severe osteoporosis where adequate fixation may not be possible, patient incompliance and excessive stress on the bone and implant, which may increase the failure rates of the implant.

What Are the Complications?

These are divided into immediate, early, late and subdivided into general and specific.

Immediate:

General: Anaesthetic risks and bleeding.

Specific: Damage to the nearby structures such as nerves, tendons and vessels, failure of the procedure due to insufficient fixation, poor reduction quality and hypersensitivity to the implant materials.

Early:

General: Deep Vein Thrombosis (DVT) and wound complications such as delayed healing and infection.

Specific: Graft extrusion, plate dislodgement and neurological symptoms such as paraesthesia.

Late:

General: Scarring.

Specific: Implant-associated infection, ossification, malunion, delayed union, pseudarthrosis, ankylosis, disarticulation, cortical necrosis and porosis.

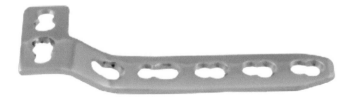

Figure 8.7   Buttress Plate. *Courtesy of Innovation Ortho Line Ltd.*

Intramedullary Nail

What Is This?

This is an intramedullary nail (Figures 8.8 and 8.9). It is a metal rod that is inserted into a long bone as an internal splint to attain a pressure-sharing mechanism thereby stabilising the fractured bone. It is inserted into the intramedullary cavity of a long bone and is secured using either screws or friction fit. Its advantages over open reduction and internal fixation include its minimally invasive nature, minimal soft tissue damage, reduced wound complication rates and fast recovery of weight-bearing ability post-operatively.

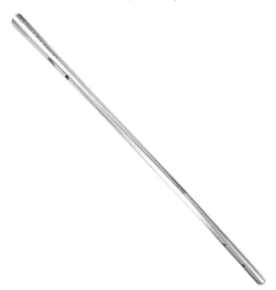

Figure 8.8   Intramedullary Nail (Femur). *Courtesy of Biomed Healthtech Ltd.*

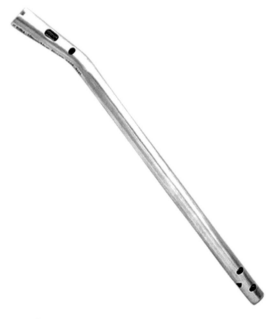

Figure 8.9   Intramedullary Nail (Tibia). *Courtesy of Biomed Healthtech Ltd.*

What Are the Indications?

Traditionally, these included mainly diaphyseal fractures of long bones including the tibia and femur. Newer designs with locking options have enabled it to extend its indications to metaphyseal fractures. It can also be used for more complicated fractures including segmental, spiral, oblique and comminuted fractures, non-union, malunion, supracondylar fractures and prophylactic treatment of impending pathological fractures.

What Are the Contraindications?

General: Active local or systemic infection. Severe osteoporosis with insufficient bone quality for implant. Hypersensitivity to the materials of the implant. General patient factors including coagulopathy and co-morbidities that would impose too high a risk to a general anaesthetic may contraindicate the procedure.

Specific: These are specific to the types of fractures and techniques used. For example, in femoral fractures, comminution extending 5 cm beyond the femoral notch would contraindicate anterograde nailing whereas fractures of the proximal femur within 5 cm of the lesser trochanter would contraindicate retrograde nailing. It is also contraindicated in paediatric open growth plate fractures.

What Are the Complications?

These are divided into immediate, early, late and are subdivided into general and specific. These can also be subdivided into site-specific complications.

Immediate:

General: Anaesthetic risks and bleeding.

Specific: Damage to the nearby structures such as nerves, tendon and vessels, implant failure due to insufficient fixation/plastic deformation/interlocking nails at very proximal or distal shaft fractures, poor reduction quality and hypersensitivity to the implant materials.

Early:

General: Deep Vein Thrombosis (DVT), pain and wound complications such as delayed healing and infection.

Specific: Graft extrusion, nail dislodgement, neurological symptoms such as paraesthesia, compartment syndrome of the thigh (femoral fractures) and avascular necrosis (AVN) of femoral head (femoral shaft nailing).

Late:

General: Scarring.

Specific: Implant-associated infection, ossification, malunion, delayed union, non-union, limb-length discrepancy, AVN of femoral head (femoral shaft nailing) and bursa formation due to soft tissue irritation (irritation from transfixing screws).

Kirschner Wire (K-Wire)

What Is This?

This is a Kirschner wire, also known as K-wire (Figure 8.10). It is a thick and sharp metal wire used to stabilise fractured bones. It also serves to align bones/fragments to a desirable position. K-wire comes in various diameters and lengths to suit the type of correction required. It can be

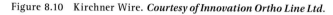

Figure 8.10   Kirchner Wire. *Courtesy of Innovation Ortho Line Ltd.*

used for a variety of procedures and a main advantage is that it can be done percutaneously under local anaesthetic. The wire can later be removed in the outpatient setting. They are particularly useful for children given the thin wires available and the ease of removal.

What Are the Indications?

They are indicated for a wide variety of procedures. These include fractures, bone reconstructions and as an adjunct in bone fixation.

Bone fracture indications include – K-wires can be used to stabilise fractures ranging from facial, phalangeal to metatarsal fractures. They can be used for either temporary or definitive fixation of fracture fragments. They can also be used as part of external fixation.

Bone reconstruction indications include – Treatment of Hallux Valgus and bunions.

As an adjunct – Acting as a guide wire/pin for the insertion of other orthopaedic implants such as cannulated screws.

What Are the Contraindications?

These are general and include: Active local or systemic infection. Hypersensitivity to the materials of the implant. Coagulopathy and co-morbidities that would impose too high a risk to a general anaesthetic may contraindicate the procedure. Patient incompliance and excessive stress on the bone and implant, which may increase the failure rates of the implant.

What Are the Complications?

These are divided into immediate, early, late and are subdivided into general and specific. These can also be subdivided into site-specific complications.

Immediate:

General: Anaesthetic risks and bleeding.

Specific: Damage to the nearby structures such as nerves, tendon and vessels, implant failure due to insufficient fixation/plastic deformation/interlocking nails at very proximal or distal shaft fractures, poor reduction quality and hypersensitivity to the implant materials.

Early:

General: Deep Vein Thrombosis (DVT), pain and wound complications such as delayed healing and infection.

Specific: Neurological symptoms such as paraesthesia, pin tract infection, pin/wire loosening and migration, loss of fixation leading to fracture movement and bending/breakage.

Late:

General: Scarring.

Specific: Pin-tract infection, implant-related infection, malunion, delayed union, non-union, bending/breakage/loosening/migration of pin/wire, over-angulation due to excessive scarring, stiffness and heterotopic ossification.

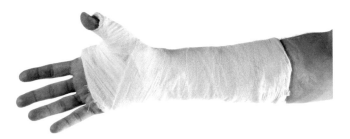

Figure 8.11   Orthopaedic Cast.

Orthopaedic Cast

What Is This?

This is an orthopaedic cast (Figure 8.11). It is a circumferential immobiliser used to support injured bones and soft tissues whilst reducing pain during the natural recovery process. Casts are custom-made to fit individuals with specific injuries. They are made from plaster or fiberglass. They are applied alongside a protective layer on the skin. It may be necessary to apply a splint before any swelling subsides and putting on a full cast.

What Are the Indications?

They are generally used for the definitive management of simple, complex and certain unstable fractures. These are wide-ranging and some common examples include non-displaced proximal/middle phalangeal shaft fractures, non-displaced/minimally displaced fractures of the distal radius, distal humeral and proximal forearm fractures, non-displaced malleolar fractures and distal metatarsal/phalangeal fractures.

They can also be used for dislocations and for soft tissue injuries when splinting is not possible.

What Are the Contraindications?

There are divided into general and specific.

General: Circumferential immobilisation is contraindicated in open fractures, shortening/angulation to an extent specific to the type of fracture, severe swelling, compartment syndrome, open wounds such as ulcers, active local infection and known ischaemia/peripheral vascular disease (PVD) and sensory defect.

Specific: Examples include tibial fractures where an initial limb shortening of >2 cm would contraindicate a cast. A fractured tibia with an intact fibula may contraindicate casting due to the potential bone deformity/fractures through compensation.

What Are the Complications?

There are divided into early and late.

Early: Ischaemia, heat injury, skin abrasions, infection, neurological injury and compartment syndrome.

Late: Chronic pain, stiffness, muscle atrophy, complex regional pain syndrome (CRPS), pressure sores, infection and neurological damage.

Further Reading

1. Boyd AS, Benjamin HJ, Asplund C. Splints and casts: Indications and methods. *Am Fam Physician.* 2009;80(5):491–9. PubMed PMID: 19725490.

2. Crawford RW, Murry DW. Total hip replacement: Indications for surgery and risk factors for failure. *Ann Rheumat Dis.* 1997;56:455–457.

3. Fitzpatrick CK, Clary CW, Cyr AJ, Maletsky LP, Rullkoetter PJ. Mechanics of post-cam engagement during simulated dynamic activity. *J Orthop Res.* 2013;31(9):1438–46. doi: 10.1002/jor.22366. Epub 2013 Apr 19. PMID: 23606458; PMCID: PMC3842834.

4. Healy WL, Iorio R, Clair AJ, Pellegrini VD, Della Valle CJ, Berend KR. Complications of total hip arthroplasty: Standardized list, definitions, and stratification developed by The Hip Society. *Clin Orthop Relat Res.* 2016;474(2):357–64. doi: 10.1007/s11999-015-4341-7. PubMed PMID: 26040966; PubMed Central PMCID: PMC4709292.

5. Mears SC. Classification and surgical approaches to hip fractures for nonsurgeons. *Clin Geriatr Med.* 2014;30(2):229–41. doi: 10.1016/j.cger.2014.01.004. Epub 2014 Mar 6. Review. PubMed PMID: 24721363.

6. Medical Advisory Secretariat. Total knee replacement: An evidence-based analysis. *Ont Health Technol Assess Ser.* 2005;5(9):1–51. Epub 2005 Jun 1. PMID: 23074478; PMCID: PMC3382388.

7. Pauyo T, Drager J, Albers A, Harvey EJ. Management of femoral neck fractures in the young patient: A critical analysis review. *World J Orthop.* 2014;5(3):204–17. doi: 10.5312/wjo.v5.i3.204. eCollection 2014 Jul 18. Review. PubMed PMID: 25035822; PubMed Central PMCID: PMC4095012.

8. Van Manen MD, Nace J, Mont MA. Management of primary knee osteoarthritis and indications for total knee arthroplasty for general practitioners. *J Am Osteopath Assoc.* 2012;112(11):709–15. Review. PubMed PMID: 23139341.

9. Webber-Jones JE, Thomas CA, Bordeaux RE Jr. The management and prevention of rigid cervical collar complications. *Orthop Nurs.* 2002;21(4):19–25; quiz 25–7. Review. PubMed PMID: 12224182.

UROLOGY

9

1) Urinary Catheter and Urometer
2) Rigid Cystoscope
3) Flexible Cystoscope

Urinary Catheter and Urometer

What Is This?

This is a urinary catheter which is lubricated and inserted through the urethral meatus and urethra into the bladder (Figures 9.1 and 9.2). It can be connected to an urometer for a more accurate measurement of urine output or to a catheter bag for easy mobilisation.

What Are the Indications?

These can be divided into investigative and therapeutic. Common investigative indications include urinary sample collection for microscopy, culture and sensitivity, and active monitoring of urine output in cases such as active bleeding and septic shock. Common therapeutic indications include acute urinary retention such as prostatism and chronic neurogenic bladder for intermittent decompression. Other therapeutic indications include clot retention in which case a 3-way catheter would be employed for a bladder washout +/− bladder irrigation. It is also used for intravesicular chemotherapy such as bacillus Calmette–Guérin (BCG) instillation.

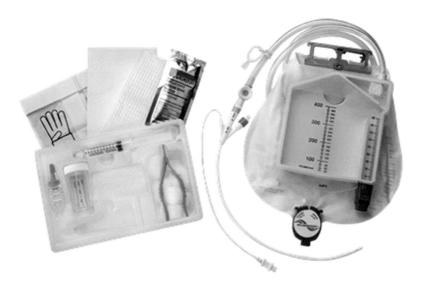

Figure 9.1 Urinary Catheter and Urometer. *Courtesy of Smiths* Medical.

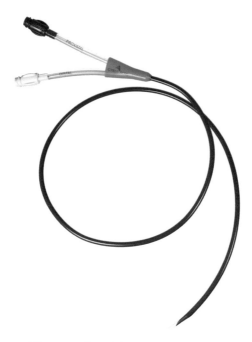

Figure 9.2   Urinary Catheter and Urometer. Copyright by Olympus Europa SE & Co. *KG.*

What Are the Contraindications?

An absolute contraindication is urethral trauma. This should be suspected in cases of pelvic injury or in any trauma case. The ATLS protocol should be followed in a trauma call. This would involve fully exposing the patient and examining the perineum, genitals and performing a digital rectal examination. Blood found at the urethral meatus, scrotal haematoma or a high-riding prostate should all raise alarm about a possible urethral tear. A retrograde urethrography should be performed in such cases to rule out any urethral injury.

Do You Know of Any Complications of Using This Device?

Common immediate complications include pain, trauma and failure of the procedure. Early complications include persistent pain and infection. Later complications may involve retrograde migration of bacteriuria leading to pyelonephritis, renal scarring and possible urethral strictures.

Rigid Cystoscope

What Is This?

This is a rigid cystoscope (Figures 9.3 through 9.5). It comes in different sizes ranging from 6 F to 27 F. Adults usually require 15 F to 25 F sizes. It is inserted into the bladder through the urethra usually under a general anaesthetic. It has a light source and a camera attached to allow for direct visualisation of the anatomical structures and any potential abnormalities. It consists of a telescope, a sheath and an obturator. The sheath consists of channels within it for the insertion of surgical instruments and passage of irrigation to distend the bladder for visual optimisation. The telescope comes with varying degrees of freedom to allow for optimised visualisation of different structures depending on anatomical locations. To minimise trauma, it is generally advised to start with the smallest cystoscope without compromise to visualisation. If clinically necessary, gradual dilatation of the urethra with Hegar dilators is performed. It offers better optical clarity over the flexible cystoscope because of the optical system and the possibility of greater irrigation flow rates.

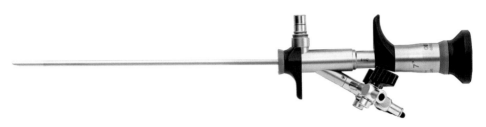

Figure 9.3   Rigid Cystoscope. *Copyright by Olympus Winter & Ibe GmbH.*

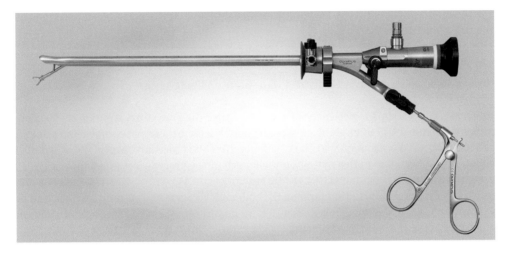

Figure 9.4   Rigid Cystoscope. *Copyright by Olympus Europa SE & Co. KG.*

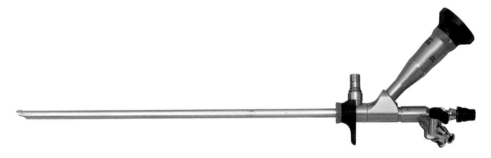

Figure 9.5   Rigid Cystoscope. *Copyright by Olympus Europa SE & Co. KG.*

What Are the Indications?

These can be divided into investigative and therapeutic.

Investigative : Haematuria, recurrent urinary tract infections (UTIs), urinary retention, urinary
   incontinence, bladder mass, prostatic symptoms, examination and biopsy of suspected
   stones/polyps/tumours/stricture.

Therapeutic : Removal of ureteric stones, removal of polyps and tumours, achieving
   haemostasis, urethral dilation, stenting after stone removal or ureteroscopy and
   treatment of urinary incontinence/overactive bladder with injections such as botulinum
   toxin. It is sometimes necessary to catheterise a patient under cystoscopy due to
   strictures.

Other investigative indications arising from other body systems: Gynaecological causes such as gynaecological tumours involving the urinary system and urinary tract injury from gynaecological and colorectal surgery.

What Are the Contraindications?

Any active urinary tract infection should preclude a cystoscopy until it is cleared. This is to avoid the risk of a urosepsis. It is common to perform a urinalysis +/– urine culture a few days before a scheduled cystoscopy. Whether prophylactic antibiotics is needed remains controversial and is beyond the scope of this book, although a recent Cochrane review found no strong evidence for its use (Zeng et al., Cochrane review, 2019). Anticoagulants may need to be stopped depending on the risk of bleeding.

What Are the Complications?

These tend to be minor and can be divided into short- and long-term.

Short-term: Most patients experience some dysuria after the procedure. Around 20–50% of patients develop a UTI or experience some form of haematuria for a few days. Occasionally, patients may need a temporary urinary catheter after the procedure, especially when bladder biopsies have been taken. Depending on the length of the procedure and amount of fluid used, transurethral resection (TUR) syndrome can occur. Very rarely, patients may develop serious complications including pulmonary embolus, myocardial infarction, stroke and deep vein thrombosis. It should also be noted that an important aspect of any hospital admission/procedure is the risk of MRSA infection.

Long-term: Iatrogenic urethral stricture.

Flexible Cystoscope

What Is This?

This is a flexible cystoscope (Figures 9.6 and 9.7). It comes in sizes ranging from 14 F to 18 F. They come in varying visual fields and deflection angles allowing the visualisation of structures depending on their locations. The optical, irrigation and instrument systems

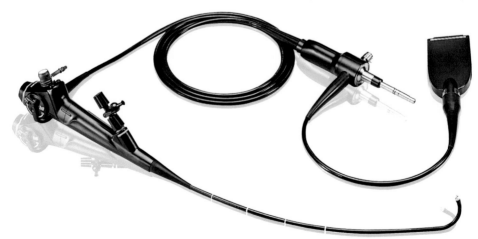

Figure 9.6   Flexible Cystoscope. *Copyright by Olympus Europa SE & Co. KG.*

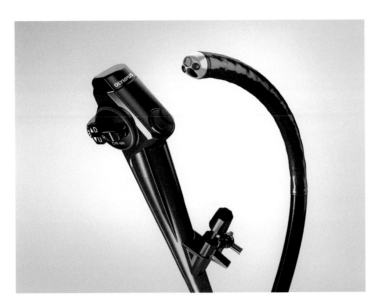

Figure 9.7   Flexible Cystoscope. *Copyright by Olympus Europa SE & Co. KG.*

all share the same working channel of the flexible cystoscope. For example, it allows the passage of an instrument to biopsy a site but does not permit simultaneous irrigation unless an adaptor is used. It offers an advantage over the rigid counterpart because of the smaller size and flexibility. These allow the procedure to be carried out in the outpatient setting with only topical anaesthetics whilst offering a wider viewing angle. It also causes less pain and discomfort for the patient than the rigid cystoscope.

What Are the Indications?

These are largely diagnostic with a few therapeutic indications these can be divided into investigative and therapeutic.

Investigative: Haematuria, recurrent urinary tract infections (UTIs), urinary retention, urinary incontinence, as well as examination and biopsy of suspected stones/polyps/tumours/stricture.

Therapeutic: Removal of stent, removal of smaller stones (+/– laser), diathermy of bleeding tissues or abnormal growths, and botulinum injections for an overactive bladder.

What Are the Contraindications?

These are similar to rigid cystoscopy. Any active urinary tract infection should preclude a cystoscopy until it is cleared. This is to avoid the risk of a urosepsis. It is common to perform a urinalysis +/– urine culture a few days before a scheduled cystoscopy. Whether prophylactic antibiotics is needed remains controversial and is beyond the scope of this book, although a recent Cochrane review found no strong evidence for its use (Zeng et al., Cochrane review, 2019).

What Are the Complications?

These are similar to but generally milder than those from a rigid cystoscopy and can again be divided into short- and long- term.

Most patients experience short-term mild dysuria and self-limiting haematuria. 1–2% of patients may develop a UTI.

Short-term: Occasionally, patients may need a temporary urinary catheter after the procedure, especially when bladder biopsies have been taken. Depending on the length of the procedure and amount of fluid used, transurethral resection (TUR) syndrome can occur. It should also be noted that an important aspect of any hospital admission/procedure is the risk of MRSA infection.

Long-term: Iatrogenic urethral stricture.

Further Reading

1. Akornor JW, Segura JW, Nehra A. General and cystoscopic procedures. *Urol Clin North Am.* 2005;32(3):319–26, vii. PubMed PMID: 16036144.
2. Engelsgjerd JS, Deibert CM. Cystoscopy. [Updated 2019 Jul 16]. StatPearls [Internet]. Treasure Island, FL: StatPearls Publishing; 2019 Jan. Available from https://www.ncbi.nlm.nih.gov/books/NBK493180/
3. Zeng S, Zhang Z, Bai Y, Sun Y, Xu C. Antimicrobial agents for preventing urinary tract infections in adults undergoing cystoscopy. *Cochr Datab System Rev* 2019;(2): CD012305. doi: 10.1002/14651858.CD012305.pub2.

MISCELLANEOUS

10

1) Nasogastric Tube
2) Anti-Embolism Stockings
3) Blood Culture Bottles
4) Fogarty Catheter
5) Coronary Angiography Balloon Catheter

Nasogastric Tube

What Is This?

This is a nasogastric (NG) tube which is inserted through the nose down the nasopharynx and oesophagus into the stomach (Figure 10.1). There are different sizes and materials depending on the purpose of the NG tube. A wider bore is used for drainage of gastric materials whereas a finer bore is used for feeding as it causes less discomfort and fewer side effects such as irritation to the nasopharynx and oesophageal erosion. Depending on the anticipated duration of enteral feeding, different materials are selected. Polyurethane and silicone are used for up to 6 weeks as they are more resistant to gastric acid erosion whereas polyvinylchloride (PVC) is less prone and only lasts up to around 2 weeks.

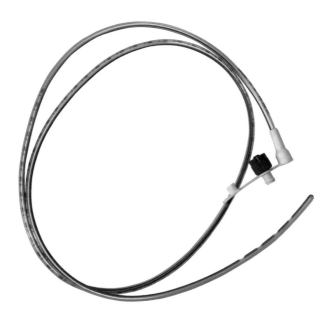

Figure 10.1   Nasogastric Tube.

What Are the Indications?

There are 2 main indications: feeding and drainage. Feeding is indicated when nutritional support is needed for the malnourished patient. It is also used when there is an obstruction in the foregut or in the case of previous head and neck surgery where swallowing is affected. Drainage/aspiration of stomach contents is needed for the decompression of intestinal obstruction as a "drip and suck" strategy.

What Are the Contraindications?

Absolute contraindications include basal skull fractures and severe facial trauma where direct trauma to the brain due to intracranial insertion is a risk. Other contraindications comprise nasal injuries, high risks of aspiration and oesophageal varices.

Do You Know of Any Complications?

Common side effects are coughing and gagging. The main complications include aspiration and trauma. Suction should be available in case of vomiting.

Anti-Embolism Stockings

What Are These?

These are anti-embolism stockings (Figure 10.2). They are worn to provide compression with a pressure gradient. They are usually worn by hospital patients to reduce the risk of DVTs. They come in different sizes and can be knee- or thigh- length.

What Are the Indications?

The main indication is the prevention of venous thromboembolism (VTE) in inpatients.

Other indications include primary chronic venous disease such as varicose veins and chronic venous insufficiency. There is evidence that the healing process of venous ulcers is expedited with compression. It can also be used in postsurgical treatment of varicose veins as a form of compression therapy though this is usually in the form of bandages.

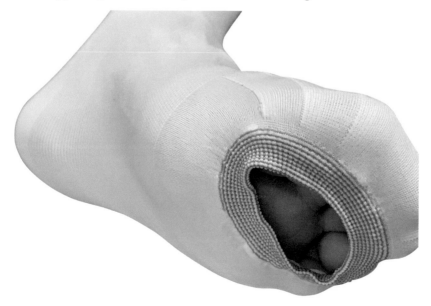

Figure 10.2   Anti-Embolism Stockings.

It is indicated in the second phase of treatment for lymphoedema as a form of maintenance therapy. It may also be used in the management of superficial thrombophlebitis.

What Are the Contraindications?

Contraindications include peripheral arterial disease (PAD), allergy to the material, severe peripheral neuropathy and local skin conditions such as recent skin graft, gangrene and infection such as cellulitis.

What Are the Complications?

These include discomfort, skin abrasions and injuries including ulcers and blisters, necrosis and worsening of PAD.

Blood Culture Bottles

What Are These?

These are blood culture bottles used for the microbiological diagnosis of aerobic and anaerobic infections (Figure 10.3). Samples are drawn from a patient's vein using the Aseptic Non-Touch Technique (ANTT). Practitioners should make sure that they fill the aerobic bottle before the anaerobic one. Bottles should be clearly labelled with the correct patient information.

What Are the Indications?

When a systemic infection is suspected.

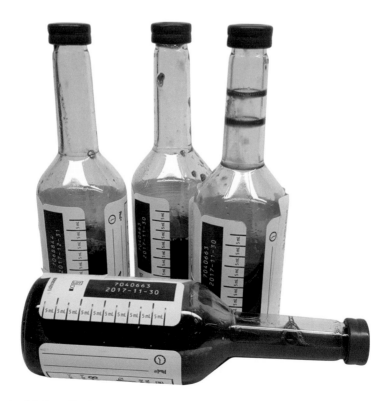

Figure 10.3   Blood Culture Bottles.

What Are the Contraindications?

Patient refusal.

What Are the Complications, If Any?

Failure of using the correct technique such as ANTT leading to contamination of the samples. Pain.

Fogarty Catheter

What Is This?

This is a Fogarty catheter, also known as a balloon embolectomy catheter (Figure 10.4). It was developed in the 1960s and was first developed for use in patients with arterial thrombi. Commonly used for lower extremity thrombi, it is usually inserted into the common femoral artery to reach the thrombus. It has an inflatable balloon at the tip which can be filled with saline to expand to the arterial wall once the tip has reached distally to the thrombus. The balloon is then retracted to the site of entry thereby removing the clot at the same time. It comes in different sizes usually

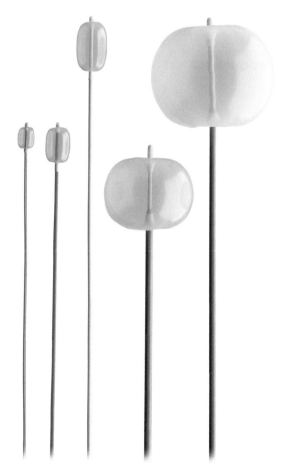

Figure 10.4   Fogarty Catheter. *Fogarty™ Occlusion Catheters, Courtesy of Edwards Lifesciences Corporation: Fogarty is a trademark of Edwards Lifesciences Corporation.*

between 2 F and 8 F. Various improvements have been made since the initial version of the Fogarty catheter. These include the Fogarty venous thrombectomy catheter, Fogarty corkscrew catheter and Fogarty Thru-Lumen Embolectomy catheter.

What Are the Indications?

The main indication is embolectomy. It was originally built for soft, fresh arterial emboli.

Later designs such as the Thru-Lumen now allow for the removal of smaller emboli/thrombi as well as fluid delivery, temporary occlusion and blood sampling. Fogarty venous thrombectomy catheters allow for the retrieval of venous thrombi. They have also been used for thromboembolic occlusion in other parts of the body including acute pulmonary embolism.

Further development of balloon catheters now also offers a variety of uses. Larger occlusion catheters (i.e. 8 F with a diameter of up to 45 mm) may be used for the occlusion control of large vessel haemorrhage including the aorta. It has also been used in as a bronchial blocker for one lung ventilation in anaesthetics to facilitate cardiothoracic/upper GI surgery. Further, it has been described in the retrieval of nasal foreign bodies.

Do You Know of Any Alternatives in Treating Thromboembolism?

Yes. Direct thrombolysis through a percutaneous catheter.

What Are the Contraindications?

These are relative. Usually patients undergo surgical thrombectomy if deemed unfit for thrombolysis. Depending on the anaesthetic technique, various contraindications exist. These include anticoagulation in patients undergoing a regional anaesthetic. Surgery for lower limb revascularisation presents high risks of cardiac mortality and may at times contraindicate such procedures especially when a general anaesthetic is required.

What Are the Complications?

These can be divided into immediate, early and late.

Immediate: Arterial perforation/rupture, pseudoaneurysm, arterio-venous (AV) fistula formation, catheter tip fracture, intima dissection and de-novo arterial thrombosis from intimal removal/damage.

Early: Arterial rupture, infection and pain.

Late: Pseudoaneurysm, accelerated atherosclerosis, diffuse arterial narrowing and AV fistula.

Coronary Angiography Balloon Catheter

What Is This?

This is a coronary angioplasty device where the balloon-tipped catheter is inserted into an artery in the groin or wrist to unblock or expand a narrowed coronary artery (Figures 10.5 and 10.6). A stent is usually implanted in the lumen to reduce the risk of recurrence.

What Are the Indications?

The main indication is coronary artery stenosis. Coronary Angioplasty can be done as an emergency or electively. Balloon angioplasty can also be used for other parts of the body. These include the carotids and other arteries in the extremities for peripheral vascular disease. Intracranial vessels can also be unblocked using this method.

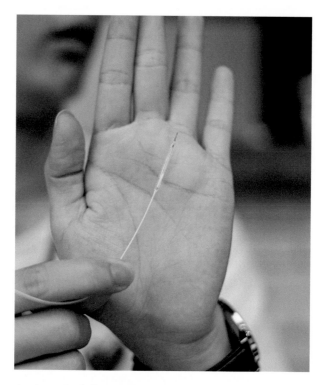

Figure 10.5   Coronary Angiography Balloon Catheter.

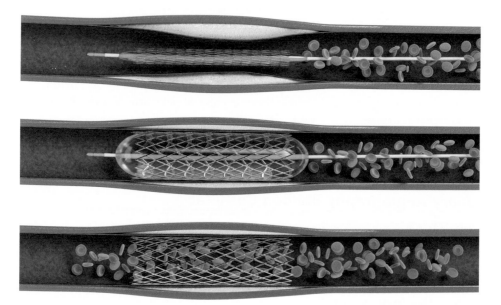

Figure 10.6   Coronary Angiography Balloon Catheter.

What Are the Contraindications?

Depending on the particular type of material used, it is contraindicated in patients with known hypersensitivity to the components. If drug-eluting stents are used, allergies to such agents may also pose risks.

After coronary artery stenting, antiplatelet with or without anticoagulation is indicated. If such therapies are contraindicated, coronary angioplasty with stenting would be contraindicated as thrombosis can occur at the stent site.

If there are lesions in the vasculature at the site of stenosis, balloon angioplasty or stenting may cause further damage and rupture, which would contraindicate the procedure.

What Are the Complications?

There are classified into immediate, early and late.

Immediate: Bleeding, pain, heart attack, stroke, coronary artery damage, arrhythmia, reperfusion injury and stent dislodgement.

Early: Contrast nephropathy, stent thrombosis and reperfusion injury.

Late: Restenosis and stent migration.

Further Reading

1. Hill B, Fogarty TJ. The use of the Fogarty catheter in 1998. *Cardiovasc Surg.* 1999;7(3):273–8. Review. PubMed PMID: 10386742.
2. Kinlay S. Management of critical limb ischemia. *Circ Cardiovasc Interv.* 2016;9(2):e001946. doi: 10.1161/CIRCINTERVENTIONS.115.001946. PubMed PMID: 26858079; PubMed Central PMCID: PMC4827334.
3. Lim CS, Davies AH. Graduated compression stockings. *CMAJ.* 2014;186(10):E391–8. doi: 10.1503/cmaj.131281. Epub 2014 Mar 3. Review. PubMed PMID: 24591279; PubMed Central PMCID: PMC4081237.
4. Manousaki E, Tsetis D, Kostas T, Katsamouris A. Endovascular treatment of a ruptured profunda femoral artery branch after Fogarty thrombectomy of a femoro-femoral crossover arterial graft: A case report and review of the literature. *Cardiovasc Intervent Radiol.* 2010;33(1):182–6. doi: 10.1007/s00270-009-9534-6. Epub 2009 Mar 17. Review. PubMed PMID: 19290575.

Index